ROBERT G. COX

The Biochemical Basis
of Neuropharmacology

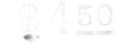

New York

Oxford University Press

London Toronto 1970

The Biochemical Basis of Neuropharmacology

JACK R. COOPER, Ph.D.

PROFESSOR OF PHARMACOLOGY

YALE UNIVERSITY SCHOOL OF MEDICINE

FLOYD E. BLOOM, M.D.

CHIEF, LABORATORY OF NEUROPHARMACOLOGY

NATIONAL INSTITUTE OF MENTAL HEALTH

WASHINGTON, D. C.

ROBERT H. ROTH, Ph.D.

ASSOCIATE PROFESSOR OF PHARMACOLOGY (PSYCHIATRY)

YALE UNIVERSITY SCHOOL OF MEDICINE

This book is dedicated to the memory of
Nicholas J. Giarman, colleague and dear friend.

Contents

The Biochemical Basis
of Neuropharmacology

1 | Introduction

WE MIGHT BROADLY DEFINE neuropharmacology as the study of drugs that affect nervous tissue. This, however, is not a practical definition since a great many drugs whose therapeutic value is extraneural can affect the nervous system. For example, the cardiotonic drug digitalis will not uncommonly produce central nervous system effects ranging from blurred vision to disorientation. For our purposes we must accordingly limit the scope of neuropharmacology to those drugs specifically employed to affect the nervous system. The domain of neuropharmacology would thus include psychotropic drugs which affect mood and behavior, anesthetics, sedatives, hypnotics, narcotics, anticonvulsants, analeptics, analgetics, and a variety of drugs that affect the autonomic nervous system. Unfortunately, these drugs which are used therapeutically are not curative. They do not eliminate the cause of the disease state but instead merely contain or control the disorder. Thus, for example, convulsive disorders for many individuals represent a life-long problem; the anticonvulsant drugs, when effective, will prevent seizures but will not alter the idiopathic seizure mechanism.

Since, with few exceptions, the precise molecular mechanism of action of these drugs is unknown, and since recitations of their absorption, metabolism, therapeutic indications, and toxic liability can be found in most textbooks of pharmacology, we have chosen to take a different approach to the subject. We will concentrate on the biochemistry and physiology of nervous tissue, emphasizing neurotransmitters, and will introduce the neuropharmacologic agents where their action is related to the subject under discussion. Thus a discussion of LSD is included in the chapter on serotonin (5-hydroxytryptamine [5-HT]) and a suggested mechanism of action of α-methyldopa in the chapter on the catecholamines.

It is not difficult to justify this focus on either real or proposed neurotransmitters since they act at junctions rather than on the events that occur with axonal conduction or within the cell body. Except for local anesthetics, which appear to interact with axonal membranes, all neuropharmacological agents whose mechanisms of action are to some extent documented seem to be involved primarily with synaptic events. This finding appears quite logical in view of the regulatory mechanisms in the transmission of nerve impulses. Whether a neuron is depolarized or hyperpolarized will depend largely on its excitatory and inhibitory synaptic inputs, and these inputs will in most cases involve neurotransmitters. It can therefore be appreciated that most neuropharmacological agents will exert their action at axo-axonic, axo-dendritic, or axo-somatic junctions. What is enormously difficult to comprehend is the contrast between the action of a drug on a simple neuron causing it either to fire or not to fire, and the wide diversity of central nervous system effects, including subtle changes in mood and behavior, which that same drug will induce.

Studying the molecular mechanisms of action of drugs affecting the nervous system, we can reason that the ultimate effect of these agents must be on ion movements, since the function of the brain is to transmit and store information, its functional unit is the neuron, and neuronal activity is expressed by ion movements across nerve membranes. It should be kept in mind, however, that the psychotropic agents, as well as drugs that affect the autonomic nervous system, appear to exert their primary effect at synapses.

The gap between our descriptive knowledge of neurotropic agents and our knowledge of molecular mechanisms of action of these drugs is wide, and it is pertinent to examine the reasons for the discrepancy. First and foremost is that to date we have been unable to locate, isolate, and characterize receptors for these various drugs. For example, although we can state that the primary site of action of barbiturates is the reticular activating system, and that structure-activity experimentation has given us some idea of the requirements, including spatial configuration, of an active barbiturate, we know very little about the physiology of the reticular activating system and nothing about the presumed attachment of a barbiturate molecule to a synapse in this system. Even more intriguing is the question why such a dramatic specificity exists in neuropharmacology, where, for example, the addition of an extra methyl group on the side chain of pentobarbital changes the compound from a hypnotic drug to a powerful convulsant drug. Even assuming that by some ingenious technique we could isolate the receptor (presumably a protein), how would we know that its properties have not changed because of its isolation from the cell? How would we prove that it was indeed the specific receptor for barbiturates? Finally, and the most difficult question, how would we relate this bit of protein to sedation and hypnosis?

Another reason we cannot explain the action of neuropharmacologic agents is that normal and abnormal neural activity at a molecular level have not been explained. And the reason for this deficiency is that biophysical research techniques and approaches of the requisite sophistication have only recently emerged.

The fact, however, that one can find compounds with a specific chemical structure to control a given pathological condition is an exciting experimental finding, since it suggests an approach that the neuropharmacologist can take to clarify normal as well as abnormal brain chemistry and physiology. The use of drugs that affect the adrenergic nervous system has, for instance, uncovered basic and hitherto unknown neural properties such as the uptake, storage, and release of the biogenic amines. The recognition of the analogy between curare poisoning in animals and myasthenia gravis in humans led to the understanding of the cholinergic neuromuscular transmission problem in myasthenia gravis and to subsequent treatment with anticholinesterases. More recently, an investigation of the action of pyrithiamine, an antimetabolite of thiamine, on isolated nerve preparations led to the discovery of the probable cause of the fatal genetic disease, subacute necrotizing encephalomyelopathy. Patients with this disease produce a compound which inhibits the synthesis in the brain of thiamine triphosphate.

The multidisciplinary aspects of pharmacology in general are particularly relevant in the field of neuropharmacology, where a "pure" neurophysiologist or neurochemist would be severely handicapped in elucidating drug action at a molecular level. The neuropharmacologist should be aware of the tools that are available for the total dissection of a biological problem. These would include techniques such as electron microscopy, freeze-etching, circular dichroism, and birefringence, as well as the classical electrophysiological and biochemical procedures. In addition, if the investigator is concerned with certain aspects of the action of psychotropic drugs, he should have some knowledge of the techniques of behavioral testing. In science, knowing what to measure is of obvious importance, but the importance of knowing how to measure it cannot be overestimated. It is for this reason that in each section of this book a critical assessment of research techniques is made. It is vital that students of neuropharmacology learn not to accept data without a severe appraisal of the procedures that were employed to obtain the results.

As already stated, our approach to neuropharmacology is by way of the basic physiology and biochemistry of nervous tissue with particular reference to neurotransmitters. The book is based on a course at Yale given to graduate and medical students. We do not intend each chapter to be a review article but rather a presentation of what we think are the important aspects of the topic. In addition, we have tried to point out serious gaps in our knowledge and to suggest possibly profitable lines of future research. Selected references, mainly recent review articles rather than original papers, are given at the end of each chapter.

2 | Cellular Foundations of Neuropharmacology

NERVE CELLS have two special properties which make them distinctive from all other cells of the body. The first is their ability to conduct bioelectric impulses over long distances without any loss of signal strength. The second, directly related to the first, is their specific input and output connections, both with other nerve cells and with innervated tissues such as muscles and glands. These connections dictate what types of information each nerve cell is to receive and what types of response it can give.

CYTOLOGY OF THE NERVE CELL

We do not need the high resolution of the electron microscope to identify several of the more characteristic structural features of the nerve cell. One of the first observations made with empirical silver impregnation stains such as the Golgi or Cajal stain was that nerve cells are heterogeneous with respect to both size and shape. (One of the confusing features of the nervous system is that each specific region of the brain and each part of each nerve cell not only has its own particular name but often has several synonymous names. So, for example, we find that the nerve cell body is also called the soma and the perikaryon—literally, the part that surrounds the nucleus).

One of the many ways of classifying nerve cells is in terms of the number of cytoplasmic processes they possess. In the simplest case, the perikaryon has but one process, called an axon; the best examples of this cell type are the sensory fibers whose perikarya occur in groups in the sensory or dorsal root ganglia. In this case, the axon conducts the signal—which was generated by the sensory receptor in the skin or other viscera—centrally through the dorsal root into the spinal cord or cranial nerve nuclei. At the next step of complexity we find neurons possessing two processes: bipolar nerve cells. The sensory receptor nerve cells of the retina, the olfactory mucosa, and the auditory nerve are of this form, as is a certain class of small nerve cells of the brain known as granule cells.

All other nerve cells tend to fall into the class known as multipolar nerve cells. While these cells possess only one axon or efferent conducting process (which may be short or long, branched or straight, and which may possess a recurrent or collateral branch which feeds back onto the same type of nerve cell from which the axon arises), the main differences are in regard to extent and size of the receptive field of the neuron, termed the dendrites or dendritic tree. In silver-stained preparations for the light microscope, the branches of the dendrites look like trees in winter time, although the branches may be long and smooth, short and complex, or bearing short spines like a cactus. It is on these dendritic branches, as well as on the cell body, where the termination of axons from other neurons makes the specialized interneuronal communication point known as the synapse, on which we will later dwell in depth.

When we examine the nerve cell with the electron microscope (Fig. 2-1) and compare it with other cell types whose biology has been well characterized, we find that in general, most nerve cells have very large nuclei in which can be seen one or more nucleoli, believed to be the sites for DNA to RNA transcription. In the cytoplasm of the perikaryon we find both free ribosomes (ribonucleoprotein sites for protein synthesis) as well as multiple cisternae of rough endoplasmic reticulum in which secretory proteins are believed to be manufactured. In addition to the free ribosomes and rough endoplasmic reticulum, we also find a specialized type of smooth endoplasmic reticulum known as

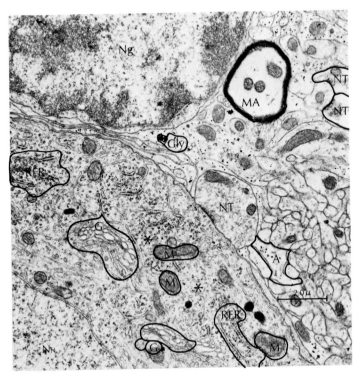

FIGURE 2-1. Low-power electron micrograph of rat cerebellar cortex. At the lower left, a large neuron can be seen. Its nucleus (Nn), two sets of Golgi apparatus (G), and areas of rough endoplasmic reticulum (RER) can be seen as well as numerous mitochondria (M) and free ribosomes (*). At upper left is the nucleus of an oligodendroglia (Ng); its cytoplasm is scant but numerous free ribosomes can be seen. One prominent nerve terminal (NT) is making specialized contact with the nerve cell. Within the nerve terminals numerous synaptic vesicles and mitochondria can be seen. One myelinated axon is shown in cross section (MA). Also visible in the neuropil are the processes of astrocytes (A) filled with glycogen granules (Gly). Two other nerve terminals (NT) are shown making specialized contacts at upper right with a dendritic spine.

the Golgi zone. In the classical secretory cycle of the pancreatic acinar cell, the Golgi zone is the site at which the secretory organelles are packaged into membrane-bound particles for transport out of the cell. Nerve cells also possess many mitochondria, the organelle specialized for oxidative phosphorylation. Mitochondria of nerves may also be able to incorporate amino acids into proteins, but the functional importance of this synthesis is as yet unexplained.

While the mitochondria occur throughout all parts of the nerve cell and its elongated processes, the rough endoplasmic reticulum is found only in the perikaryon and in the dendrites. The dendrites and the axons both exhibit microtubules, elongated tubular objects 240 Å in diameter whose long axis runs throughout the extent of the axon or dendrite. These microtubules are identical in fine structure to similar organelles found in other cell types in which their function is believed to be cellular support. Although this may be their main function in the elongated cytoplasmic processes of the nerve cell, some scientists have proposed that the microtubules may serve as directional guides for the cytoplasmic transport of cellular ingredients from the cell body to more distal parts of the cell. Microtubules with the same structure and amino acid composition as neuronal microtubules function in the nucleus during mitosis to separate the DNA components of the chromosomes. This process can be blocked by the drug colchicine, which breaks up the subunits of the microtubules. Radioactive colchicine can be shown to bind specifically to the microtubules of the nerve cell and to block transport of many neuronal constituents down the axon.

In addition to mitochondria and microtubules, axons also exhibit structures called neurofilaments. Biochemically, the neurofilaments appear to be composed of the same sub-units as the microtubules although they are organized into a much smaller (100 Å) fibrous structure. Generally, axons which have large numbers of microtubules have very few filaments, and vice versa. Small (i.e. narrow) axons tend to have microtubules but few neurofilaments. Large axons may have many neurofilaments but few microtubules. In some cases the neurofilaments may extend into the nerve ending, where they tend to form a ring-like configuration around the external perimeter of the nerve-ending axoplasm. Except for the fact that the neurofilaments can be stained by silver and probably account for the so-called neurofibrils of classical light microscopy, no specific functions for neurofilaments have yet been uncovered.

The Synapse

The last specialized structural features of the neuron we shall discuss are the contents of the nerve ending and the characteristics of the specialized contact which has been identified as the site of functional interneuronal communication. As the axon approaches the site of its termination it exhibits structural features not found more proximally (Fig. 2-2). Most striking is the occurrence of large numbers of microvesicles, which have been dubbed synaptic vesicles. These structures tend to be spherical in shape, with diameters varying between 200 and 1200 Å. Depending upon the type of fixation used, the vesicles may exhibit one or more types of internal electron-opaque granularities; this cytochemical characteristic is related to certain endogenous small molecules considered to be potential synaptic transmitting substances (see Chapters 4 and 5). The nerve endings also exhibit mitochondria, but never exhibit microtubules unless the nerve ending belongs to the class of axons possessing several accumulations of synaptic vesicles along their terminal passage. Each of these endings forms a specialized contact with one or more dendritic branches before the ultimate termination. Such endings are known as *en passant* terminals. In this sense, the term "nerve terminal" or "nerve ending" connotes more a functional transmitting site than a structural blind alley.

Electron micrographs of synaptic regions in the central nervous system reveal a specialized contact zone between the axonal nerve ending and the postsynaptic structure. This specialized contact zone is composed of presumed proteinaceous material lin-

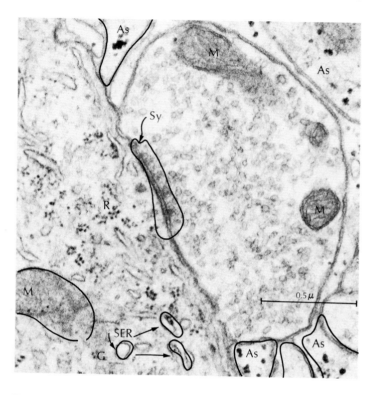

FIGURE 2-2. High-power view of the same nerve ending seen in Fig. 1. At this magnification the synaptic vesicles can be seen more clearly, as can the zone of specialized contact (Sy). Astrocyte processes containing glycogen (As) can be seen as well as smooth endoplasmic reticulum (SER) and free ribosomes (R) within the cytoplasm of the nerve cell. Note that only about half of the contact between the nerve terminal and the nerve cell membrane exhibits the specialized zone of contact.

ing the intracellular portions of the pre- and postsynaptic membranes and filling the synaptic cleft between the apposed cell surfaces. Such types of specialized contacts are a general form of the specialized cell contacts seen between many types of cell derived from the embryonic ectoderm, of which the nerve cell is but one. However, the specialized contact between neurons is polarized: that is, the presynaptic terminal intracellular material is composed of interrupted presynaptic dense projections measuring about 500-700 Å in diameter and separated from each other by distances of 300-400 Å. This material may be present only to bind specific presynaptic nerve endings permanently to specific postsynaptic cell sites. Alternatively, the specialized contact zone could assist in the efficiency of transmission and could constitute one potential method for modulating synaptic transmission in terms of discharge frequency. This is a subject upon which much future research can be expected.

Functional Interpretations from Cytology

If we were to try to infer the functions of a neuron from the foregoing catalogue of its cellular machinery, we would be entitled to the following assumptions. Despite wide variations in cell shape, size, and volume, most nerve cells possess large amounts of unattached ribosomes, presumably for the synthesis of intracellular materials such as enzymes and structural macromolecules. However, the cell body is also filled with varying quantities of rough endoplasmic reticulum and smooth endoplasmic reticulum indicative of cells that package synthetic material for transcellular secretion. Thus, we anticipate the neuron to be a dynamic secretory cell with broad synthetic capabilities.

While organelles with such synthesizing capabilities characterize both the dendrite and cell body cytoplasm, they are never found within the axon. Since the axon possesses no apparent synthetic capacity of its own, other mechanisms have had to be developed to explain the way in which the axon can maintain its vitality. One such proposal is that the cell body synthesizes all the required macromolecules for the axon and that a process of cytoplasmic flow carries them from the cell body down the axon. This theory of axoplasmic flow has been substantiated by studies involving actual physical barriers to axonal flow and by labeling proteins in the cell body to time their rates of migration toward the periphery. Such studies have indicated that the flow rates may vary from as little as one-tenth of a millimeter per day to as much as many centimeters in an hour, depending upon the organelle or metabolite used as a tracer.

Glia

A second element in the maintenance of the axon's integrity depends on a type of cell known as neuroglia, which we have not yet discussed. There are two main types of neuroglia. The first is called the fibrous astrocyte, a descriptive term based on its star-like shape in the light microscope and on the fibrous nature of its cytoplasmic organelles, which can be seen in both light and electron microscopy. The astrocyte is found mainly in regions of axons and dendrites and tends to surround or contact the adventitial surface of blood vessels. Functions such as insulation (between conducting surfaces) and organization (to surround and separate functional units of nerve endings and dendrites) have been empirically attributed to the astrocyte, mainly on the basis of its structural characteristics.

The second type of neuroglia is known as the oligodendrocyte. It is called the satellite cell when it occurs close to nerve cell bodies, and the Schwann cell when it occurs in the peripheral nervous system. The cytoplasm of the oligodendrocyte is characterized by rough endoplasmic reticulum but its most prominent characteristic is the enclosure of concentric layers of its own surface membrane around the axon. These concentric layers come together so closely that the oligodendrocyte cytoplasm is completely squeezed out and the original internal surfaces of the membrane become fused, presenting the ring-like appearance of the myelin sheath in cross section (Fig. 2-1). Along the course of an axon, which may be many centimeters in length, many oligodendrocytes are required to constitute its myelin sheath. At the boundary between adjacent portions of the axon covered by separate oligodendrocytes, there is an uncovered axonal portion known as the node of Ranvier.

Many central axons and certain elements of the peripheral autonomic nervous system do not possess myelin sheaths. Even these axons, however, are not bare and exposed to the extracellular fluid, but rather they are enclosed within single invaginations of the oligodendrocyte surface membrane. Because of this close relationship between the conducting portions of the nerve cell, its axon, and the oligodendrocyte, it is easy to see the origin of the proposition that the oligodendrocyte may contribute to the nurture of the nerve cell. While this idea may be correct, no evidence is yet available. Clearly, the glia are incapable of supporting the axon when it has been severed from the cell body, for example, by trauma or by surgically induced lesioning. This incapacity is fortuitous for neuroscientists, since one of the chief methods of defining nerve circuits within the brain has been the staining of degenerating axons following brain lesions.

Brain Permeability Barriers

While the unique cytological characteristics of neurons and glia are sufficient to establish the complex intercellular relationships of the brain, there is yet another histophysiologic concept to consider. Numerous chemical substances pass from the bloodstream into the brain at rates which are far slower than for entry into all other organs in the body. There are similar slow rates of transport between the cerebrospinal fluid and the brain, although there is no good standard in other organs against which to compare this latter movement.

These permeability barriers appear to be the end result of numerous contributing factors which present diffusional obstacles to chemicals on the basis of molecular size, charge, solubility, and specific carrier systems. The difficulty has not been in establishing the existence of these barriers, but rather in determining their mechanisms. When the relatively small protein (MW = 43,000) horseradish peroxidase is injected intravenously into mice, its location within the tissue can be demonstrated histochemically with the electron microscope. As opposed to the easy transvascular movement of this substance across muscle capillaries, in brain the peroxidase molecule is unable to penetrate through the continuous layer of vascular endothelial cells. The endothelial cells of brain capillaries differ from those of other tissue such as muscle and heart in that the intercellular zones of membrane apposition are much more highly developed in the brain, and are virtually continuous along all surfaces of these cells. Furthermore, cerebral vascular endothelial cells show a distinct lack of pinocytotic vesicles which have been related to transvascular carrier systems of both large and small molecules.

Since the enzyme marker can neither go through or between the endothelial cells, an operationally defined barrier exists. Whether the same barrier is also applicable to highly charged lipophobic small molecules cannot be determined from these observations. As neuropharmacologists, what concerns us most here are the factors which retard the entrance of these smaller molecules, such as norepinephrine and serotonin, their amino acid precursors, or drugs which affect the catabolism or synthesis of these two neurotransmitters. For these substances, the poorly conceived and minimally studied barriers may be tentatively considered as solvent partitions across the vasculature, since many such molecules when permitted entry via the cerebrospinal fluid, are able to diffuse widely through the extracellular spaces of the brain. While these extracellular spaces were long interpreted as exceedingly small on the basis of electron micrographs, we now know that the lack of space was an artifact due to swelling of astrocytes during fixation. Thus, once a substance can enter the perivascular extracellular spaces of the brain, it is likely to encounter few barriers which would prevent it from migrating between cells—presumably along concentration gradients, but possibly moved by specific carriers—to reach those neurons or glia capable of incorporating it, responding to it, or metabolizing it.

The barriers are not one-way, since those same substances which find it difficult to get into the brain also find it exceedingly difficult to leave. Thus, when the monoamines are increased in concentration by the blocking of their catabolic pathways (see Chapter 5), the high levels of amine persist until the inhibiting agents are metabolized or excreted. One such route is the "acid transport" system by which the choroid plexus and/or brain parenchymal cells actively secrete acid catabolites. This step can be blocked by the drug probenecid, resulting in increased brain and CSF catabolites of the amines.

Since the precise nature of these barriers can still not be formulated, the student would be wise to avoid the "great wall of China" concept and lean toward the possibility of a series of variously placed, progressively selective filtration sites, which discriminate substances on the basis of several molecular characteristics.

BIOELECTRIC PROPERTIES OF THE NERVE CELL

With these structural details as a background, we can now turn to the best-known feature of the nerve cell, namely, its bioelectric property. However, even for an introductory presentation such as this, we must understand certain basic concepts of the physical phenomena of electricity in order to have a working knowledge of the bioelectric characteristics of living cells.

The initial concept to grasp is that of a difference in potential existing within a charged field, as occurs when charged particles are separated and prevented from randomly redistributing themselves. When a potential difference exists, the amount of charge per unit of time which will flow between the two sites (that is, current flow) depends upon the resistance separating them. If the resistance tends to zero, no net current will flow since no potential difference can exist in the absence of a measurable resistance. If the resistance is extremely high, only a minimal current will flow and that will be proportional to the electromotive force or potential difference between the two sites. The relationship between voltage, current, and resistance is the famous Ohm's law, expressed as:

FIGURE 2-3. At the top is shown a hypothetical neuron (Nl) receiving a single excitatory pathway (E) and a single inhibitory pathway (I). A stimulating electrode (S) has been placed on the nerve cell's axon; microelectrode 1 is extracellular to nerve cell 1, while microelectrode 2 is in the cell body, and microelectrode 3 is in its nerve terminal. Microelectrode 4 is recording from within postsynaptic cell 2. The potentials and current, recorded by each of these electrodes, are being compared through a "black box" of electronics with a distant extracellular grounded electrode, and displayed on an oscilloscope screen. When the cell is resting and the electrode is on the outside of the cell, no potential difference is observed (1). In the resting state, electrode 2 records a steady potential difference between inside and outside of approximately minus 50 millivolts (2). While recording from electrode 2 and stimulating the inhibitory pathway, the membrane potential is hyperpolarized during the inhibitory postsynaptic potential (2 + I). When recording from electrode 2 and stimulating the excitatory pathway, a subthreshold stimulus (St) produced an excitatory postsynaptic potential indicated by a brief depolarization of the resting membrane potential (2 + E). When the excitatory effects are sufficient to reach threshold (T), an action potential is generated which reverses the inside negativity to inside positivity (2 + E). On the lower scale, potentials recorded by electrodes 3 and 4 are compared on the same time-base following axonal stimulation of nerve cell 1. The point of stimulus is seen as an electrical artifact at point S. The action potential generated at the nerve terminal occurs after a finite lag period due to the conduction time (c) of the axon between the stimulating electrode and the nerve terminal. The action potential in the nerve ending does not directly influence postsynaptic cell 2 until after the transmitter has been liberated and can react with nerve cell 2's membrane, causing the excitatory postsynaptic potential indicated by the dotted line. The time between the beginning of the action potential recorded by microelectrode 3 and the excitatory postsynaptic potential recorded by electrode 4 (A) is the time required for excitation secretion coupling in the nerve terminal and the liberation of sufficient transmitter to produce effects on nerve cell 2.

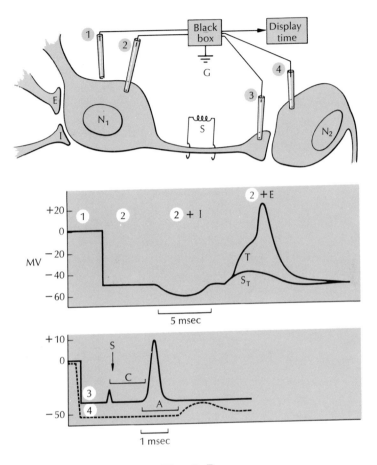

$$V = I \cdot R.$$

When we come to the measurement of the electrical properties of living cells, these basic physical laws apply, but with one
exception. The pioneer electrobiologists, who did their work before the discovery and definition of the electron, developed a
convention for the flow of charges based not on the electron but
on the flow of positive charges. Therefore, since in biological systems the flow of charges is not carried by electrons but by ions,

the direction of flow is expressed in terms of movement of positive charges. To analyze the electrical potentials of a living system, we use small electrodes (a microprobe for detecting current flow or potential), electronic amplifiers for increasing the size of the current or potential, and oscilloscopes or polygraphs for displaying the potentials observed against a time base.

Membrane Potentials

If we take two electrodes and place them on the outside of a living cell or tissue, we will find little, if any, difference in potential. However, if we injure a cell so as to break its membrane or insert one ultra-fine electrode across the membrane, we will find a potential difference such that the inside of the cell is 50 or more millivolts negative with respect to the extracellular electrode (Fig. 2-3). This transmembrane potential difference is found in almost all types of living cells in which it has been sought; such a membrane is said to be electrically polarized. By passing negative ions into the cell through the microelectrode (or extracting cations), the inside can be made more negative (hyperpolarized). If positive current is applied to the inside of the cell the transmembrane potential difference is decreased, and the potential is said to be depolarized. The potential difference across the membrane of most living cells can be accounted for by the relative distribution of the intracellular and extracellular ions.

The extracellular fluid is particularly rich in sodium and relatively low in potassium. Inside the cell, the cytoplasm is relatively high in potassium content and very low in sodium. While the membrane of the cell permits potassium ions (K^+) to flow back and forth with relative freedom, it resists the movement of the sodium ions (Na^+) from the extracellular fluid to the inside of the cell. Since the potassium ions can cross the membrane they tend to flow along the concentration gradient—which is highest inside the cell. Potassium diffusion out of the cell leaves a relative negative charge behind due to the negative charges of the macromolecular proteins. As the negative charge inside the cell begins to build up, the further diffusion of potassium from inside to out-side is retarded. Eventually an equilibrium point will be reached which is proportional to certain physical constants and to the relative concentrations of intracellular and extracellular potassium and chloride ions. These features apply generally, not only to nerve and muscle cells but also to red blood cells, gland cells, and other cells large enough to have their transmembrane potential measured.

Membrane Leaks and Pumps

When the nerve cell or muscle fiber can be placed in a dish and transmembrane potential recordings made, the relation be-tween the membrane potential and external potassium concentra-tion can be directly tested by exchanging the extracellular fluid for artificial solutions of varying potassium concentration. When this experiment is performed on muscle cells, we find that the membrane potential bears a linear relationship to the external po-tassium concentration at normal to high potassium concentrations, but deviates from this linear relationship when the external potas-sium concentration is less than normal. To account for this dis-crepancy we must now re-examine an earlier statement. While the plasma membranes of nerve and muscle cells and other types of polarized cells are relatively impermeable to the flow of so-dium ions along the high concentration gradient from extracel-lular to intracellular, they are not completely impermeable. With radioisotope experiments it can be established that a certain amount of sodium leaks into the resting cell from outside. The amount of measurable sodium leakage into the cell occurs at a rate sufficient to double the intracellular sodium concentration in approximately one hour if there were not some opposing process to maintain the relatively low intracellular sodium concentration. The process which continuously maintains the low intracellular sodium concentration is known as active sodium transport, or col-loquially as the "sodium pump." This pump mechanism ejects sodium from the inside of the cell against the high concentration and electrical gradients forcing it in. However, the "pump" does not handle sodium exclusively but requires the presence of extracellular potassium, so that when a sodium ion is ejected from the cell, a potassium ion is incorporated into the cell.

When the external potassium concentration is near normal, the transmembrane potential, which is based mainly on potassium concentration differences, behaves as if there were actually more extracellular potassium than really exists. This is because the sodium-potassium exchange mechanism elevates the amount of potassium coming into the cell. Remember that potassium permeability is relatively high and that potassium will tend to diffuse out of the cell because of its concentration gradient but to diffuse into the cell because of charge attraction. Therefore, two factors operate to drive potassium into the cell in the presence of relatively low external potassium concentration: (1) the electrical gradient across the membrane and (2) the sodium-potassium pump mechanism. The latter system could be considered "electrogenic" since at low external K^+ concentrations it modifies the electrical status of the muscle membrane. Other metabolic pumps operate simply to exchange cationic species across the membrane and are "nonelectrogenic." The relative "electrogenicity" of a pump may depend on the ratio of the exchange cations (i.e. 1 : 1 or 2 : 1, or 3 : 2). The pump is immediately dependent upon metabolic energy and can be blocked by several metabolic poisons such as dinitrophenol and the rapid acting cardiac glycoside, ouabain.

The Uniqueness of Nerve

All that we have said regarding the transmembrane ionic distributions applies equally as well to the red blood cell membrane as to the nerve membrane. Thus, the possession of a transmembrane potential difference is not sufficient to account for the bioelectric properties of the nerve cell. The essential difference between the red blood cell and the nerve cell can be brought out by applying depolarizing currents across the membrane. When the red blood cell membrane is depolarized, the difference in potential across the cell passively follows the imposed polarization. However, when a nerve cell membrane, such as the giant axon of an invertebrate, is depolarized from a resting value of approximately −70 millivolts to approximately −10 to −15 millivolts, an explosive self-limiting process occurs by which the transmembrane potential is reduced not merely to zero but overshoots zero, so that the inside of the membrane now becomes positive with respect to the outside. This overshoot may extend for 10 to 30 millivolts in the positive direction. Because of this explosive response to an electrical depolarization the nerve membrane is said to be electrically excitable, and the resultant explosion is known as the action potential.

Analysis of Action Potentials

In an elegant series of now classical pioneering experiments, Hodgkin, Huxley, and Katz were able to analyze the various ionic steps responsible for the action potential. When the cell begins to depolarize from stimulation current, the current flow across the membrane is carried by potassium. As the membrane becomes more depolarized, the conductance across the membrane to sodium (conductance is the inverse expression of resistance) increases and more sodium flows into the cell along its electrical and concentration gradients. As sodium flows in, the membrane becomes more and more depolarized which further increases the conductance to sodium, further depolarizing the membrane at a greater rate. This self-perpetuating process continues until the sodium ions reach their equilibrium distribution, which should be proportional to the original extracellular and intracellular concentrations of sodium.

However, the peak of the action potential does not quite attain the equilibrium potential predicted on the basis of transmembrane sodium concentrations because of a second phase of events. The electrical process which leads to the rapidly increasing conductance to sodium also further increases, after a slight delay, the transmembrane conductance to potassium, whose flow then also begins to increase along its concentration gradient, that is, from inside to outside the cell. This process restricts the height of the reversal potential since it tends to maintain the inside negativity of the cell and also begins to reduce the membrane conductance to sodium, thus making the action potential a self-limiting phenomena. In most nerve axons, the action potential lasts for approximately 0.2 to 0.5 milliseconds, depending on the type of fiber and the temperature in which it is measured.

Once the axon has reached threshold, the action potential will be propagated at a rate which is proportional to the diameter of the axon and which is further accelerated by the presence of the glial myelin sheaths, which restrict the active conducting points to the node of Ranvier. As mentioned above, these are the only sites on the myelinated axons at which the axonal membrane is directly exposed to the extracellular fluid and thus are the only sites at which transmembrane ionic flows can take place. Therefore, instead of the action potential propagating from minutely contiguous sites of the membrane, the action potential in the myelinated axon leaps from node to node. This saltatory conduction is consequently much more rapid.

The threshold level for an all-or-none action potential is also inversely proportional to the diameter of the axon: large myelinated axons respond to low values of imposed stimulating current, whereas fine and unmyelinated axons require much greater depolarizing currents. Local anesthetics appear to act by blocking activation of the sodium conductance preventing depolarization.

Once threshold has been reached, a complete action potential will be developed unless it occurs too quickly after a preceding action potential, during the so-called refractory phase. This phase varies for different types of excitable nerve and muscle cells and appears to be related to the activation process increasing sodium conductance, a phenomenon which has a finite cycling period; that is, the membrane cannot be reactivated before a finite interval of time has occurred. Potassium conductance increases with the action potential after a delay and lasts longer than the activation of sodium conductance. This results in a prolonged phase of after-hyperpolarization due to the continued redistribution of potassium from inside to outside the membrane. If the axonal membrane is artificially maintained at a transmembrane potential equal to the potassium equilibrium potential, no after-hyperpolarization can be seen.

Junctional Transmission

While these ionic mechanisms appear to account adequately for the phenomena occurring in the propogation of action potential down an axon, they do not *per se* explain what happens when the action potential reaches the nerve ending. At the nerve ending the membrane of the axon is separated from the membrane of the postjunctional nerve cell, muscle, or gland by an intercellular space of 50-200 Å (Fig. 2-2). In those cases in which an electrode can be placed in both the terminal axon and the postsynaptic cell, depolarization of the nerve terminal does not usually result in a direct and instantaneous shift in the transmembrane potential of the postsynaptic element. Thus, the junctional site seldom appears to have the properties of direct electrical excitability described above for the axon.

Axons versus Junctions

Junctional or synaptic transmission varies in certain important characteristics from axonal transmission. Firstly, impulses travel in only one direction across synaptic or junctional sites. In this regard the junction can be said to be a rectifier or valve permitting only one direction of flow. In the axon, impulses can be made to travel in the proper (or orthodromic) direction from receptor to axon terminal; however, if the distal end of an axon is stimulated and recordings made from its cell body, the action potential will also travel backward up the axon. This is known as antidromic activation.

We have already mentioned that the depolarization of the postjunctional cell is separated in time by at least 0.1 to 0.2 msec from activity in the presynaptic terminal. This transmission delay time cannot be accounted for simply on the basis of the electrical resistance and capacitance between the junctional elements and suggests that a separate and nonelectrical process occurs at the transmission site. No such delays are seen with conduction down the axon (see above). Transmission across junctional sites has finite temporal limits and the postsynaptic element cannot usually follow the presynaptic element at stimulation rates higher than 100/sec. Junctional sites are also extremely sensitive to drugs and hypoxia. On the other hand, axonal transmission can follow stimulation rates as high as 1500/sec at which time they are limited only by the relative refractory period of the axon.

A final distinguishing characteristic between junctional and axonal transmission is that subthreshold presynaptic stimuli can combine in time to lead to a threshold stimulus and produce firing. This is due to the fact that subthreshold potential changes have a prolonged electrotonic spread; second subthreshold stimulus can have a cumulative effect upon the residua of a previous declining subthreshold stimulus. On the other hand, in axons, action potentials are either all-or-none, and no such temporal summation can be demonstrated. Temporal summation can result in the postsynaptic cell continuing to discharge for several msec after the stimulation of the presynaptic element has stopped. Firing in the axon begins and ends with the imposed stimulation, and normally no after-discharges occur.

Postsynaptic Potentials

With the advent of microelectrode techniques for recording the transmembrane potential of nerve cells *in vivo*, it was possible to determine the effects of stimulation of nerve pathways which had previously been shown to cause either excitation or inhibition of synaptic transmission. From just such studies Eccles and his colleagues observed that subthreshold excitatory stimuli would produce postsynaptic potentials with time durations of 2 to 20 msec. The excitatory postsynaptic potentials could algebraically summate both with the excitatory and inhibitory postsynaptic potentials. Most importantly, the duration of these postsynaptic potentials was longer than could be accounted for on the basis of electrical activity in the preterminal axon or on the electrotonic conductive properties of the postsynaptic membrane (Fig. 2-3). This latter observation combined with the fact that synaptic sites are not directly electrically excitable provides the conclusive evidence that central synaptic transmission must be chemical: the prolonged time course is compatible with a rapidly released chemical transmitter whose time course of action is terminated by local enzymes, diffusion, and re-uptake by the nerve ending.

By such experiments it was possible to work out the basic ionic mechanisms for inhibitory and excitatory postsynaptic potentials. When an excitatory pathway is stimulated, the presynaptic element liberates an excitatory transmitter which is able to activate the ionic conductance of the postsynaptic membrane. This leads to a generalized increase in all transmembrane ionic conductances, forcing the membrane to move toward the sodium equilibrium potential; in the resting state, as has already been discussed, the membrane resides near the potassium equilibrium potential. The approach to the sodium equilibrium potential results in depolarization, and if this is sufficient to reach the threshold for adjacent electrically excitable portions of the cell membrane, an all-or-none action potential will result. If the resultant depolarization is insufficient to reach firing threshold, the cell may still discharge if additional excitatory postsynaptic potentials summate adequately before the first excitatory potential has disappeared.

The inhibitory postsynaptic potential resulting from the stimulation of an inhibitory pathway to the postsynaptic cell has been explained in terms of the fact that inhibitory transmitter is able selectively to activate conductance for chloride, resulting in an inward diffusion of this ion and a further hyperpolarization of the membrane. This counter-balances the excitatory postsynaptic potentials.

Because the sites of synaptic or junctional transmission are electrically inexcitable, the postsynaptic membrane potential can be maintained at various levels by applying current through intracellular electrodes and changing the intracellular concentrations of various ions. By such maneuvers, it is possible to poise the membrane at or near the so-called equilibrium potentials for each of the ionic species and to determine the ionic species whose equilibrium potential corresponds to the conductance change caused by the synaptic transmitter. This is the most molecular test for the identification of actions of a synaptic transmitter substance. (However, certain objections can be raised to this test in terms of those nerve endings making junctional contacts on distal portions of the dendritic tree. Here, the postsynaptic potentials may be incompletely transmitted to the cell body in which the recording electrode is placed.)

Slow Postsynaptic Potentials

Most of the postsynaptic potentials described by Eccles and his colleagues were relatively short, usually 20 msec or less and appear to result from passive changes in ionic conductance. Recently postsynaptic potentials of slow onset and several seconds' duration have been described (Fig. 2-3), both of a hyperpolarizing nature and of a depolarizing nature. While such prolonged postsynaptic potentials could be due either to a prolonged release of transmitter or to a persistence of the transmitter at postsynaptic receptor sites, there is substantial support for the possibility that slow postsynaptic potentials could also be caused by the specific stimulation of metabolically coupled electrogenic pump mechanisms in the postsynaptic membrane. These "pump-activated" synaptic junctions are not associated with changes in ionic conductance and obviously would have no "equilibrium potential." However, they should be sensitive to metabolic poisons. Slow postsynaptic potentials may be extremely important in the intermediate (i.e. between brief and permanent) term regulation of cellular activity. These potentials are the type of event by which specific facilitation (or depression) of conduction could modulate activity of certain nerve circuits (i.e. memory—see Chapter 9).

Transmitter Secretion

We have already seen that the cellular machinery of the neuron suggests it functions as a secretory cell. The secretion of synaptic transmitters is the activity-locked expression of neuronal activity induced by the depolarization of the nerve terminal. Recently, it has been possible to separate the excitation-secretion coupling process of the presynaptic terminal into at least two distinct phases. This has been made possible through an analysis of the action of the puffer fish poison tetrodotoxin, which blocks the electrical excitation of the axon but does not block the release of transmitter substance from the depolarized nerve terminal. The best of such experiments have been performed in the giant synaptic junctions of the squid stellate ganglion, in which the nerve terminals are large enough to be impaled by recording and stimulating microelectrodes, and recording from the post-synaptic ganglion neurons. In this case, when tetrodotoxin blocks conduction of action potentials down the axon, electrical depolarization of the presynaptic terminal still results in the appearance of an excitatory postsynaptic potential in the ganglion neuron. Since the action of tetrodotoxin appears to be relatively selective for the early activation of increase in Na^+ conductance, the excitation secretion may be coupled more closely to the process causing the delayed increase in K^+ conductance. However, Ca^{++} must also be present in sufficient concentration or no release will occur. Although the long-distance conducting portions of mammalian central neurons appear to be electrically excitable, the points at which nerve cells communicate now appear to be exclusively chemical.

An Approach to Neuropharmacological Analysis

You can now see that the business of analyzing bioelectrical potentials can be very complicated even when restricted to the changes in single neurons or in small portions of contiguous neurons. But if we restrict our examination of centrally-active drugs to analyses of effects on single cells we can ask rather precise questions. For example, does drug "X" act on resting membrane potential or resistance, on an electrogenic pump, or on the sodium-or potassium-activation phase of the action potential, or does it act by blocking or modulating the effects of junctional transmission between two specific groups of cells.

Unfortunately, both for us and for the literature, we have had these precise electrophysiological tools for less than ten years. Therefore earlier neuropharmacologists were required to examine effects of the drug on populations of nerve cells. This was usually done in one of two ways. Large macroelectrodes were employed to measure the potential difference between one brain region and another. These electroencephalograms reflect mainly the moment to moment algebraic and spatial summations of slow synaptic potentials, and almost none of their electrical activity is due to actual action potentials generated by individual neurons (unit discharges). A second type of analysis was based on evoked responses, in which macroelectrodes recorded the potential changes occurring when a gross sensory stimulation (such as a flash of light or a quick sound) was delivered. Changes in recordings from cortical or subcortical sites along the sensory pathway were then sought during the action of a drug. While we can criticize the technical and interpretative shortcomings of such methods of central drug analysis, these methods were able to reflect the population response of a group of neurons to a drug, something which single unit analysis can do only after many single recordings are collated.

Approaches

If, as modern-day neuropharmacologists, we are chiefly concerned with uncovering the mechanisms of action of drugs in the brain, there are several avenues along which we can organize our attack. We could choose to examine the way in which drugs influence the perception of sensory signals by higher intergrative centers of the brain; this is compatible with a single neuron and ionic conductance type of analysis, such as how do drugs affect inhibitory postsynaptic potentials. Drugs which cause convulsions, such as strychnine, have been analyzed in this respect, but all types of inhibitory postsynaptic potential are not affected by strychnine.

A second basic approach would be to use both macroelectrodes and microelectrodes to compare the drug response of single units and populations of units in the same brain region. However, this approach is clearly limited unless we understand the intimate functional relations between the multiple types of cells found even within one region of the brain.

A third approach is also possible. We could choose to separate the effects of drugs between those affecting generation of the action potential and its propagation, and those acting on junctional transmission. For this type of analysis, we must identify the chemical synaptic transmitter for the junctions to be studied. Many of the interpretative problems already alluded to can be attacked through this approach. Thus, as you may expect, there is likely to be more than one type of excitatory and inhibitory transmitter substance, and a convulsant drug might affect the response to one type of inhibitory transmitter without affecting another. Moreover, a drug might have specific regional effects in the brain if it could affect a unique synaptic transmitter there. In fact, using this approach it might be possible to find drug effects not directly reflected in electrical activity at all, but related more to the catabolic or anabolic systems maintaining the required functional levels of transmitter. We shall conclude this chapter by considering the techniques for identifying the synaptic transmitter for particular synaptic connections. The chapters which follow are organized to present in detail our current understanding of putative central neurotransmitter substances.

IDENTIFICATION OF SYNAPTIC TRANSMITTERS

How then, do we identify the substance released by nerve endings? The entire concept of chemical junctional transmission arose from the classical experiments of Otto Loewi, who demonstrated chemical transmission by transferring the ventricular fluid of a stimulated frog heart onto a nonstimulated frog heart, thereby showing that the effects of the nerve stimulus on the first heart were reproduced by the chemical activity of the solution flowing onto the second heart. Since the phenomenon of chemical transmission originated from studies of peripheral autonomic organs, these peripheral junctions have become convenient model systems for central neuropharmacological analysis.

Certain interdependent criteria have been developed to identify junctional transmitters. By common-sense analysis, one would suspect that the most important criterion would be that a substance suspected of being a junctional transmitter must be demonstrated to be released from the prejunctional nerve endings when the nerve fibers are selectively stimulated. This criterion was relatively easily satisfied for isolated autonomic organs where only one or at most two nerve trunks enter the tissue, and the whole system can be isolated in an organ bath. In the central nervous system, however, satisfaction of this criterion presumes: (a) that the proper nerve trunk or set of nerve axons can be selectively stimulated and (b) that release of the transmitter can be detected in the amounts released by single nerve endings after one action potential. This last subcriterion is necessary since we wish to restrict our analysis to the first set of activated nerve endings and not examine the substances released by the secondary and tertiary interneurons in the chain, some of which might reside quite close to the primary endings. The biggest problem with this criterion in the brain, however, is the lack of a method for detecting release which does not in itself destroy the functional and structural integrity of the region of the brain being analyzed. Such techniques as internally perfused cannulae or surface suction cups are chemically at the same level of resolution as the evoked potential and the cortical electroencephalogram: each of these methods records the resultant activity of thousands if not millions of nerve endings and synaptic potentials. Release has also been studied in brain slices incubated in "physiological buffer solutions" *in vitro*. While these techniques can demonstrate the effects of very large electrical depolarizing potentials, the relationship of a brain slice to the living brain remains to be determined.

Localization

Because it is difficult, if not impossible, to identify the substance released from single nerve endings by selective stimulation, the next-best evidence might be to prove that a suspected synaptic transmitter resides in the presynaptic terminal of our selected nerve pathway. Normally, we would expect that the enzymes for synthesizing and catabolizing this substance should also be in the vicinity of this nerve ending, if not actually part of the nerve ending cellular machinery. For satisfaction of this criterion, several types of specific cytochemical methods for both light microscopy and electron microscopy have been developed. More commonly employed is the biochemical population approach, analyzing the regional concentrations of suspected synaptic transmitter substances. However, presence *per se* indicates neither release-ability nor neuro-effectiveness (e.g. acetylcholine in the nerve-free placenta or serotonin in the enterochromaffin cell).

Synaptic Mimicry: Drug Injections

A third criterion arising from the peripheral autonomic nervous system analysis is that the suspected exogenous substance mimics the action of the transmitter released by nerve stimulation. In most pharmacological studies of the nervous system, drugs are administered intravascularly or onto one of the external or internal surfaces of the brain. The substances could also be directly injected into a given region of the brain although the resultant structural damage would have to be controlled and the target verified histologically. The analysis of the effects of drugs given by each of these various gross routes of administration is quite complex.

We know that diffusional barriers selectively retard the entrance from the bloodstream of many types of molecules into the brain. These barriers have been demonstrated for most of the suspected central synaptic agents. In addition, we suspect that extracellular catabolic enzymes could destroy the transmitter as it diffuses to the postulated site of action. A further complicating aspect of these gross methods of administration is that the interval of time from the administration of the agent to the recording of the response is usually quite long (several seconds to several minutes) in comparison with the millisecond intervals required for junctional transmission. The delay in response further reduces the likelihood of detecting the primary site of action on one of a chain of neurons.

Microelectrophoresis

The student will now realize how important it is to have methods of drug administration equal in sophistication to those with which the electrical phenomena are detected. The most practical micromethod of drug administration yet devised is based upon the principle of electrophoresis. Micropipettes are constructed in which one or several barrels contain an ionized solution of the chemical substance under investigation. The substance is applied by appropriately directing the current flow. The microelectrophoretic technique, when applied with controls to rule out the effects of pH, electrical current, and diffusion of the drug to neighboring neurons, has been able to overcome the major limitations of the classical neuropharmacological techniques. Frequently, a multiple-barreled electrode is constructed from which one records the spontaneous extracellular discharges of single neurons while other attached pipettes are utilized to apply drugs. One can also construct an intracellular microelectrode glued to an extracellular drug-containing multi-electrode, so that the transmembrane effects of these suspected transmitter agents can be compared with the effects of nerve pathway stimulation. The intracellular electrode can also be used to poise the relative polarization of the membrane and let us detect whether the applied suspected transmitter and that released by nerve stimulation cause the membrane to approach identical ionic equilibrium potentials.

Pharmacology of Synaptic Effects

The fourth criterion for identification of a synaptic transmitter requires identical pharmacological effects of drugs potentiating or blocking postsynaptic responses to both the neurally released and administered samples. Because the pharmacological effects are often not identical (most "classical" blocking agents are extrapolated to brain from effects on peripheral autonomic organs), this fourth criterion is often satisfied indirectly with a series of circumstantial pieces of data. Recently, with the advent of drugs blocking the synthesis of specific transmitter agents, the pharmacology for certain families of transmitters has been improved.

The application of drugs has thus far been evaluated on four types of single-cell activity. The response of the cell to the putative transmitter agent and to the neurally released substance can be compared with respect to effects on: (a) spontaneous activity, (b) orthodromic synaptically evoked activity, (c) antidromic activity, and (d) induced effects caused by excitatory or inhibitory substances applied from another barrel of the micropipette. These techniques have been most successful when applied to large neurons, whose selected afferent pathways can be stimulated and the transmembrane effects specifically analyzed. However, when the unit recording techniques are applied to the mammalian brain, visualization and selection of the neuron under investigation are almost impossible. Although we can generally select a relatively specific brain region in which to insert the microelectrode assembly, we must utilize electrophysiological criteria for its identification. We must also depend upon geometrical attributes of the nerve cell to encounter its electrical activity as the electrode is navigated by blind mechanical means through the brain. Our ability to encounter cells in the brain depends partly on the size

FIGURE 2-4. Ten steps in the synaptic transmission process are indicated in this idealized synaptic connection. Step 1 is transport down the axon. Step 2 is the electrically excitable membrane of the axon. Step 3 involves the organelles and enzymes present in the nerve terminal for synthesizing, storing, and releasing the transmitter, as well as for the process of active re-uptake. Step 4 includes the enzymes present in the extracellular space and within the glia for catabolizing excess transmitter released from nerve terminals. Step 5 is the postsynaptic receptor which triggers the response of the postsynaptic cell to the transmitter. Step 6 shows the organelles within the postsynaptic cells which respond to the receptor trigger. Step 7 is the interaction between genetic mechanism of the postsynaptic nerve cell and its influences on the cytoplasmic organelles which respond to transmitter action. Step 8 includes the possible "plastic" steps modifiable by events at the specialized synaptic contact zone. Step 9 includes the electrical portion of the nerve cell membrane which, in response to the various transmitters, is able to integrate the postsynaptic potentials and produce an action potential. Step 10 is the continuation of the information transmission by which this postsynaptic cell sends an action potential down its axon.

---

and type of the electrode assembly we use, partly on the size and spontaneous activity of the cell we are approaching, and partly on the surgical or chemical means by which we have prepared the animal (namely, presence or absence of anesthesia, homeostatic levels of blood pressure and tissue oxygen and carbon dioxide). Even with very fine microelectrodes, the analysis does not take place in a completely undisturbed system since many connections must be broken by the physical maneuvering of the electrode. The leakage of cytoplasmic constituents, including potential transmitter agents and metabolic enzymes, can only be considered as part of the background artifact of the system.

THE STEPS OF SYNAPTIC TRANSMISSION

Let us now conclude this chapter by examining in a summary fashion the mechanisms of presumed synaptic transmission

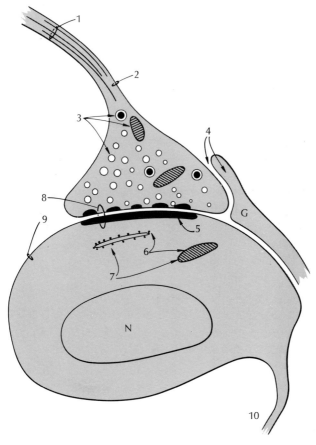

for the mammalian central nervous system. Each step in such transmission constitutes one of the potential sites of central drug action (Fig. 2-4). A natural or imposed stimulus activates an all-or-none action potential in an axon by depolarizing its transmembrane potential above the threshold level. The action potential propagates in an unattentuated manner to the nerve terminal where the depolarization activates a mobilization process allowing the specific transmitter for the junction to act upon the postsynaptic cell. From companion biochemical experiments (to be described in the next chapters), the transmitter substance is believed to be stored within the microvesicles or synaptic vesicles seen in nerve endings by electron microscopy. In certain types of nerve junctions, miniature postsynaptic potentials can be seen in the absence of conducted presynaptic action potentials. These miniature potentials have a quantatized effect on the postsynaptic membrane in that occasional potentials are statistical multiples of the smallest measurable potentials. The biophysical quanta have been related to the synaptic vesicles, although the proof for this relationship is still circumstantial.

When the transmitter is released from its storage site by the presynaptic action potential, the effects on the postsynaptic cells cause either excitatory or inhibitory postsynaptic potentials, depending upon the nature of the postsynaptic cell's receptor for the particular transmitter agent. If sufficient excitatory postsynaptic potentials summate temporally from various inputs onto the cell, the postsynaptic cell will integrate these potentials and give off its own all-or-nothing action potential, which is then transmitted to each of its own axon terminals, and the process continues.

Akert, K., H. Moor, K. Pfenninger, and C. Sandri (1969). Contributions of new impregnation methods and freeze etching to the problems of synaptic fine suture. *Progr. Brain Res. 31*, 203.

Bloom, F. E. (1968). Electrophysiological pharmacology of single nerve cells. In *Psychopharmacology, A Review of Progress* (D. H. Efron, ed.) p. 355. Government Printing Office, Washington, D.C.

Bodian, D. (1967). Neurons, circuits and neuroglia. In *The Neurosciences—A Study Program* (F. O. Schmitt, G. C. Quarton, and T. Melnechuk, eds.), p. 6. Rockefeller Univ. Press, New York.

Brodie, B. B., H. Kurz, and L. S. Schanker (1960). The importance of dissociation constant and lipid solubility in influencing the passage of drugs into the cerebrospinal fluid. *J. Pharmacol. 130*, 20.

Eccles, J. C. (1964). *The Physiology of Synapses*. Academic Press, New York.

Grundfest, H. (1967). Synaptic and ephaptic transmission. In *The Neuro-Sciences—A Study Program (op. cit.)*, p. 347.

Hodgkin, A. L., and A. F. Huxley (1952). Currents carried by sodium and potassium ions through the membrane of the giant axon of *Loligo. J. Physiol. 116:* 449.

Hodgkin, A. L., A. F. Huxley, and B. Katz (1949). Ionic currents underlying activity in the giant axon of the squid. *Arch. Sci. Physiol. 3:* 129.

Katz, B. (1966). *Nerve, Muscle and Synapse*. McGraw-Hill, New York.

Lajtha, A., and D. H. Ford (1968). Brain barrier systems. *Progr. Brain. Res. 29*, 1.

Loewi, O. (1921). Uber humorale Ubertragbarkeit der Herznervenwirkung. *Pflugers Arch. ges. Physiol. 189:* 239.

Salmoiraghi, G. C., and F. E. Bloom (1964). Pharmacology of individual neurons. *Science 144,* 493.

3 | Biochemistry of the Central Nervous System

BEFORE ENTERING into a discussion of the biochemistry of nervous tissue, it is of some importance to describe the kinds of preparations of neural tissue that have been employed in neurochemical studies as well as the techniques available for the assay of enzymes and substrates. There is no universal preparation that is satisfactory for all types of biochemical analyses. Indeed, some of our currently accepted neurochemical information derives from preparations of unknown composition that consequently contain unknown contributions of glial or Schwann cell tissue.

TECHNIQUES AND PREPARATIONS

The various techniques and preparations used in neurochemical studies may be listed as follows, starting with whole animal preparations and progressing to simpler neural elements:

(a) *Arterio-venous differences.* Pioneered by Schmidt in 1928, this technique involves sampling arterial blood for O_2 and CO_2 (generally the carotid artery is used) and simultaneously measuring the concentration of these gases in venous blood leaving the brain via the jugular vein. On occasion, glucose and a variety of metabolites such as pyruvate and lactate have also been determined. From these studies it was found that the respiratory quotient is usually very close to one, indicating that carbohydrate is the primary energy source of the brain.

(b) *Brain lesions.* Using stereotactic localization, relatively discrete areas of brain tissue can be destroyed. With this technique, Heller and Harvey have recently studied the monoamine pathways of the forebrain.

(c) *Whole brain perfusion.* In this procedure, involving extensive and literally death-defying surgery, arterial and venous blood vessels in the head region of the cat, other than vessels that are cannulated for the perfusion, are occluded, and defibrinated blood or an artificial solution containing erythrocytes and albumin is perfused. This technique, exploited mainly by Geiger and his associates, is not widely used, not only because of the difficult operative procedure but also because of the abnormal EEG and abnormal values of glucose utilization. These findings cast some doubt on the usefulness of this preparation.

(d) *Perfusion of the spinal cord.* By cannulating the vertebral canal of intact bull frogs (*Rana catesbiana*), Burgen, Angelucci, and others have developed a simple preparation of central nervous system tissue. These investigators stimulated the cord by stimulating the sciatic nerve and measured the increased efflux of a variety of neuroactive substances.

(e) *Perfusion of peripheral nervous tissue.* As discussed in Chapter 4, the bulk of our current information on the turnover of acetylcholine (ACh) in nervous tissue comes from the studies of MacIntosh and his colleagues on the perfused superior cervical ganglion of the cat. The metabolism of the perfused excised organ has also been extensively studied by Larrabee, who investigated the effects of barbiturates on oxygen consumption and more recently phospholipid turnover. Numerous investigations have utilized perfused isolated peripheral nerves such as the sciatic or the vagus in studying the effect of drugs on conduction.

(f) *Cortical cups.* Plastic rings mounted on an exposed surface of the cerebral hemispheres or cerebellum have been used to collect putative neurotransmitters. Compounds such as ACh seep into the enclosed area after electrical stimulation or the administration of drugs to the animal. The technique has been refined by Mitchell and by Pepeu.

(g) *Regional cannulae.* Developed by Feldberg, who studied effects of injected catecholamines on body temperature, cannulae with two cylinders have now been devised, one cylinder for injecting material and one for withdrawing it. Both intraventricular and intracerebral cannulae are available.

(h) *Tissue culture.* Murray and co-workers have successfully cultured a variety of neural elements, including the superior cervical ganglion and spinal neurons which have been used to test neuropharmacologic agents.

(i) *Hand dissection.* By the use of a dissecting microscope, neuronal fragments (shorn of dendritic branches) have been isolated by Roots and Johnson, Edstrom, Hydén, and Giacobini, among others. Lowry in particular has developed techniques for handling excised nervous tissue, including the development of a quartz fiber fishpole balance that can weigh amounts of tissue as little as 0.0001 μg.

(j) *Centrifugal "dissection."* Brain fractions enriched in neuronal and glial elements have been separated by Rose using Ficoll density gradient centrifugation. This technique has been questioned because uncontaminated neuronal and glial fractions have not been reproduced in other laboratories. Norton has recently developed a much more satisfactory procedure.

(k) *Cerebral cortical slices.* The ease of preparing brain slices coupled with the demonstration in McIlwain's laboratory that this preparation yields a propagated action potential makes tissue slices a popular tool for many biochemical investigations. Since most of the cells are intact it is unnecessary to fortify the preparation with coenzymes or other cofactors. Cut surfaces are an advantage in that added substrates may penetrate easily but a disadvantage in that leakage of materials out of the slice will also occur.

(l) *Homogenates.* The technique of disrupting cells is an obvious prelude to the isolation of enzymes and of subcellular organelles.

(m) *Nerve ending particles and synaptic vesicles.* Developed independently by De Robertis and Whittaker, these preparations derive from a sucrose density gradient centrifugation of a crude mitochondrial fraction from brain. The centrifugation results in several distinct bands of material that can be identified by electron microscopy as myelin and membrane fragments, pinched-off nerve ending particles with attached postsynaptic membrane, and mitochondria. The nerve ending particles (sometimes called synaptosomes) may be ruptured by osmotic shock to release synaptic vesicles, the putative containers of neurotransmitters. Often overlooked in the isolation of synaptosomes is the fact that the heterogeneity of brain precludes a knowledge of just what percentage of the synaptosomes are cholinergic, noradrenergic, serotonergic, etc. In addition it is difficult to determine if the properties of these particles have changed during the isolation procedure.

ASSAYS

With respect to the determination of substances of biochemical interest, neurotransmitters may be assayed quantitatively using either bioassay or chemical procedures as outlined in appropriate chapters. Substrates and enzymes are determined with a variety of physico-chemical techniques. In roughly increasing order of sensitivity, these would be manometry, colorimetry, spectrophotometry, gas-liquid chromatography, microgasometry, fluorometry, and radioactivity.

Fluorometric procedures should be singled out in particular because of their inherent specificity and sensitivity. In this regard, Lowry and his colleagues have imaginatively utilized the native and inducible fluorescence of the pyridine nucleotides as first described by Greengard. By coupling substrates and enzymes to the ultimate oxidation or reduction of pyridine nucleotides, these investigators have measured as little as 10^{-19} moles of substrate. By way of illustration one might consider the following coupled system:

$$\text{glucose} + \text{ATP} \xrightarrow{\text{Hexokinase}} \text{glucose-6-phosphate} + \text{ADP}$$

$$\text{glucose-6-phosphate} + \text{NADP} \xrightarrow{\text{glucose-6-phosphate dehydrogenase}} \text{6-phosphogluconate} + \text{NADPH} + \text{H}^+$$

Sum: glucose + ATP + NADP $\longrightarrow$ 6-phosphogluconate + ADP + NADPH + H^+

It is readily apparent that, utilizing these reactions, one can determine the concentration of glucose, ATP, or the activity of hexokinase merely by making it rate-limiting in the system and measuring NADPH either spectrophotometrically or fluorometrically, depending on the sensitivity that is required.

Neurochemical Studies

With this introduction into methodology it is now proper to ask what has been measured with respect to brain biochemistry and whether the acquired information illuminates the unique function of the brain.

One approach to this subject is to go through the litany of the Embden-Meyerhof glycolytic pathway, the tricarboxylic acid cycle, the pentose phosphate shunt, and the biosynthetic and metabolic pathways of carbohydrates, lipids, nucleic acids, and proteins. All of these enzyme systems occur in brain and have been studied in more or less detail, but qualitatively there is nothing of striking import to distinguish these enzyme activities in nervous tissue from their activity in extraneuronal tissue. For example, the synthesis of ATP from glycolysis and oxidative phosphorylation appears not to be fundamentally different in brain than in other tissues and does nothing to illuminate the brain as a specialized organ. In particular, if one recalls the diversity as well as the specificity of effects of neurotropic agents, it is difficult to see the relevance of such a universal and basic mechanism as energy production in a discussion of neuropharmacology. Unless neuropharmacological agents had a peculiar affinity for nervous tissue one would not expect to encounter such a specificity among these agents if they directly inhibited glycolysis or oxidative phosphorylation. More logically, the mechanism of action of these agents might be anticipated to lie in their ability ultimately to affect neurotransmitters. This could be primarily by displacement of the neurotransmitters or by affecting the synthesis, release, catabolism, storage, or re-uptake of transmitters or by altering ion movement in axons.

To state the obvious, then, since the brain is an organ which transmits and stores information, it seems most profitable in discussing the biochemistry of the brain to look at enzyme systems and substrates that may contribute to this specialization. In other words, if one were asked to identify biochemically a piece of tissue as brain, what would one determine? Accepting this challenge, we can now proceed to list the types of compounds and enzyme systems which can be used to elucidate the biochemical uniqueness of brain as well as to point out profitable future lines of experimental investigations:

(A) *Compounds with demonstrated electrophysiological activity.*

(B) *Compounds and enzyme systems that either occur only in the CNS or whose concentration in the brain is extraordinarily high compared with that of other tissues.* A concentration of > 3 mM has been arbitrarily chosen as a cutoff point.

(C) *Compounds in which a change in concentration in*

brain has been shown to correlate with a change in the behavioral state of the animal.

The composite flow sheet of Figure 3-1 covers to a large extent the listings above. The arrows are not intended to imply direct conversions but merely precursor relationships. For convenience, compounds in Group A are in capital letters; compounds in Group B are enclosed in blocks, and compounds in Group C are underlined.

The graph properly begins with glucose, because in brain, in contrast to other tissues, virtually everything except essential amino acids is derived from this substrate. For example, when labeled glucose is incubated with brain cortical slices, labeled aspartate and glutamate appear within a few minutes after the addition of the glucose to the flasks. The same occurs *in vivo* as well as in brain perfusion experiments.

The knowledge that glucose is under normal conditions the primary if not the sole substrate of the brain *in vivo* derives from two experimental findings. First, as stated earlier, in measuring A-V differences in O_2 and CO_2 in the blood going through the brain, a respiratory quotient of 1 was obtained, indicating that the oxidation of carbohydrates rather than amino acids or fatty acids is the primary source of energy. Further, when the A-V differences of glucose, glutamate, lactate, and pyruvate were determined, the only compound removed in large amounts from the arterial blood was glucose, and the only product that was released in large quantities was CO_2. The second line of evidence implicating glucose derives from experiments on the hypoglycemia induced either by hepatectomy or by the administration of insulin. In these experiments the fall in blood glucose correlated with a cerebral dysfunction that ranged from mild behavioral impairment to coma. This CNS effect can be completely reversed by the administration of glucose, maltose, or mannose, the latter two being converted to glucose. It is not reversed by lactate, pyruvate, or glutamate (perhaps because these agents do not penetrate the blood-brain barrier at a high enough rate). In insulin coma, with its concomitant low cerebral metabolic rate, there is enough glucose and glycogen to last about 90 minutes; then other cerebral metabolites are utilized. This calculation correlates with the observation that in insulin coma irreversible damage occurs after 90 minutes despite the subsequent administration of glucose. This irreversibility may be due to the fact that vital amino acids and lipids are utilized in an attempt to maintain cerebral metabolism.

The first step in glucose metabolism involves a phosphorylation by ATP (via the enzyme hexokinase) to form glucose-6-phosphate. About 90 per cent of this phosphate ester is metabolized through the well-known Embden-Meyerhof glycolytic pathway and about 10 per cent is oxidized via the pentose phosphate cycle. This latter system, sometimes referred to as the hexose monophosphate shunt, does not lead directly to ATP synthesis, as is the case with glycolysis or oxidative phosphorylation. Instead, it appears to function primarily in providing reduced nicotinamide adenine dinucleotide phosphate (NADPH), vital in lipid biosynthesis, and the pentose phosphates that are required in the *de novo* synthesis of nucleotides.

The Embden-Meyerhof pathway leads to triose phosphates which are involved in the synthesis of lipids. The high concentration of lipids is a unique feature of brain since about 50 per cent of the dry weight of brain is lipid compared with 6 to 20 per cent in other organs of the body. In further contrast to other tissues, there is only free cholesterol and virtually no cholesterol esters in brain.

In addition to cholesterol, brain lipids include glycerides and sphingolipids of very complex composition. The composition of some of these compounds is shown in Table 3-1. Protein-lipid complexes are also found in nervous tissue and are referred to as proteolipids or lipoproteins, depending on the physical characteristics of the molecule. Phosphatidopeptides have also been reported in the brain. Although the chemistry of brain lipids is fairly well known and much is being learned currently of the synthesis and catabolism of lipids, the function of these compounds is still unclear. What is clear is that most lipids serve as structural components, either in myelin or in membranes of the various cellular organelles, and exhibit a slow turnover. However,

TABLE 3.1. Lipid Structures

Basic Structure	R_1	R_2	X	Compound
CH_2-O-R_1 R_2-O-CH $\quad\quad\quad O$ $CH_2-O-P-O-X$ $\quad\quad\quad O-$ glycerophosphate	fatty acid	fatty acid	$CH_2CH_2NH_2$	phosphatidylethanol-amine
	fatty acid	fatty acid	$CH_2CH_2N^+(CH_3)_3$	phosphatidylcholine
	fatty acid	fatty acid	(inositol ring structure)	phosphatidylinositol (di- and triphospho-inositides have phosphate on position 4 and 5)
	H	OPO_3H	H	cardiolipin (diphosphatidyl glycerol

Basic Structure	Addition	Compound
$CH_3(CH_2)_{12}CH=$ $CH(OH)CH(NH_2)CH_2OH$ sphingosine	fatty acid	ceramide
	fatty acid, phosphorylcholine	sphingomyelin
	galactose	psychosine
	galactose, fatty acid	cerebroside
	galactose, fatty acid, sulfate	sulfatide
	glucose, galactose, fatty acid, N-acetylneuraminic acid, N-acetylgalactosamine	ganglioside

$$HO_2C-\overset{O}{\overset{\|}{C}}-CH_2-CHOH-\overset{H}{\underset{NH-\underset{\|}{\overset{}{C}}-CH_3}{\overset{|}{C}}}-(CHOH)_3-CH_2OH$$

N-acetylneuraminic acid (sialic acid)

a metabolic function for phosphoinositides has been suggested by several investigators. Among phosphatides, the inositol phosphatides show the most rapid incorporation of $P^{32}O_4$, both *in vivo* and *in vitro;* in addition this turnover in the superior cervical ganglion is stimulated either by the addition of ACh or by preganglionic stimulation.

Although the function of the complex lipids is unknown, their implication in certain genetic types of mental retardation known as the cerebral lipidoses is well documented. Thus, for example, in Tay-Sachs disease there is an accumulation of gangliosides, in Gaucher's disease the cerebroside content of the brain rises, and in Niemann-Pick disease there is an accumulation of both sphingomyelin and gangliosides. It is also known that in demyelinating diseases the cerebroside and sphingomyelin content of the brain declines and that there is a formation of cholesterol esters.

Continuing with the scheme in Figure 3-1, the offshoot giving rise to ACh, glycine, and prostaglandins will be dealt with where these neurotransmitters, real or putative, are discussed in the subsequent chapters.

Glutamate is the next compound we encounter in Figure 3-1 which fulfills our criteria for neuropharmacological interest. Besides its obvious utility in the brain as an energy source in coupled phosphorylation and as an amino acid for protein synthesis, glutamate has four other functions. It serves as:

1. a "detoxifying" substrate trapping NH_3 to form glutamine;
2. the precursor of γ-aminobutyric acid (GABA);
3. one of the amino acids in glutathione;
4. a "universal" excitatory amino acid.

The possible neurotransmitter roles of glutamate and of GABA will be discussed in Chapter 7. Also to be discussed in that chapter is the "GABA shunt," a sequence of reactions unique to brain, in which glutamate functions catalytically to produce succinate from α-oxoglutarate without invoking α-oxoglutarate dehydrogenase. In its role in the pathways sketched in Figure 3-1, GABA condenses with choline to form γ-aminobutyrylcholine,

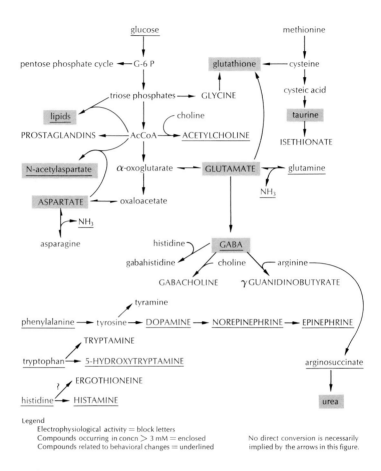

FIGURE 3-1. Various interrelationships among compounds of neuropharmacological interest.

with arginine to yield γ-guanidinobutyrate, and with histidine to produce γ-aminobutyrylhistidine. γ-Aminobutyrylcholine and γ-guanidobutyrate have been shown to exert an inhibitory effect on evoked cortical potentials. However, the high concentrations that were necessary to evoke a response makes their physiological function suspect. Virtually nothing is known about the possible physiological role of γ-aminobutyrylhistidine.

The relationship between ammonia levels in the brain and convulsions has been demonstrated in a variety of experimental procedures. Although the cerebral origin of endogenous ammonia production is still unclear, the role of glutamate and glutamine synthetase in ammonia disposal is well established. Thus the infusion of ammonium salts into dogs results in an increased level of cerebral glutamine. Glutamine levels are presumably regulated by diffusion of the compound into the general circulation to the kidney where glutaminase would remove ammonia. The ammonia would be eliminated either as a cation or via the urea cycle. Under normal conditions glutamine might be regarded as a storehouse for glutamate; the observation that glutaminase is an allosteric enzyme that is activated by phosphate, ammonia, and nucleoside triphosphates and inhibited by glutamate suggests that the conversion of glutamine to glutamate is under fine metabolic control.

Glutathione is a tripeptide consisting of glutamic acid, cysteine, and glycine. Although glutathione has been known for about forty years, its function still remains elusive. It does serve as the coenzyme for the conversion of methylglyoxal to lactic acid by glyoxylase, and the isomerization of maleylacetoacetate to fumarylacetoacetate, but these reactions are not considered important enough to explain its high concentration in brain. Rather, speculation on the role of the tripeptide has always revolved around its oxidation and reduction. The oxidized or disulfide form of glutathione is rapidly reduced by a specific NADPH-dependent glutathione reductase in brain; the reaction is essentially irreversible. Glutathione may be oxidized either in maintaining other cerebral constituents in a reduced form or in its destruction of hydrogen peroxide that is formed in oxidase reactions, e.g. xanthine oxidase. This cycle would then be:

1. $R\text{-}S\text{-}S\text{-}R + 2GSH \longrightarrow 2RSH + G\text{-}S\text{-}S\text{-}G$

or

$H_2O_2 + 2GSH \longrightarrow 2H_2O + G\text{-}S\text{-}S\text{-}G$

2. $G\text{-}S\text{-}S\text{-}G + NADPH + H^+ \longrightarrow 2GSH + NADP^+$

The NADPH would presumably be provided by the activity of glucose-6-phosphate dehydrogenase and 6-phosphogluconate dehydrogenase in the pentose phosphate cycle.

We would not be *au courant* if we failed to describe a final neuropharmacological implication of glutamate, the Chinese restaurant syndrome. Some individuals experience painful reactions after eating Chinese food. The syndrome has been traced to the large amount of monosodium glutamate used in some recipes.

The transamination of glutamate with oxaloacetate leads to aspartate. Although in some invertebrates this amino acid serves as an organic anion reservoir, in mammalian tissue its role appears to be metabolic. Like glutamate, aspartate has central excitatory activity on iontophoretic application, can serve as a readily available energy source, and can also trap ammonia to form asparagine. Aspartic acid is a requisite in *de novo* nucleotide synthesis and in the arginosuccinic acid synthetase reaction in brain (see below).

In the presence of acetyl CoA and a specific enzyme from brain, aspartate forms N-acetylaspartate, a very intriguing compound. N-acetylaspartate is of interest in that (a) next to glutamic acid it is the amino acid or derivative in highest concentration in the brain and (b) except for trace amounts in spinal roots it occurs only in the brain. Although in weanling animals the acetyl group can contribute to lipid biosynthesis in the brain, in adults the compound is believed to be somewhat inert metabolically. Attempts to label N-acetylaspartate by injecting radioactive precursors or *in vitro* by incubating cerebral slices with labeled glucose or aspartate have yielded only trace amounts of radioactive N-acetylaspartate. However, when labeled N-acetylaspartate is incubated with cerebral slices a small amount of N-acetylaspartyl peptides is formed. Although the level of N-acetylaspartate remains remarkably constant (about 5.4 mM) in the face of insulin shock or the administration of analeptics, sedatives, or anesthetic agents, certain drugs that appear to be related to 5-hydroxytryptamine (5-HT) produce a change in the concentration of this amino acid derivative in brain. Thus, the administration of iproniazid or 5-hydroxytryptophan (5-HTP) but not dihydroxyphenylanine (DOPA) to mice causes a rise in the level of acetylaspartate whereas LSD-25 produces a fall. The change in the level of acetylaspartate, however, follows by several hours the change in 5-HT levels in the brain so that this relationship is apparently indirect. From these drug studies the half-life of N-acetylaspartic acid in brain has been calculated to be about 12 ± 3 hours.

The fact that N-acetylaspartate has been shown to be localized in cell cytoplasm, that it has an apparently long turnover time, and that as a dicarboxylic acid it contributes approximately 11 meq of anion/kg of brain, raises the possibility that acetylaspartate functions solely as an anion to help defray the so-called "anion deficit" that exists.

Arising from the metabolism of the essential amino acid methionine are cysteic acid and taurine. This pair is reminiscent electrophysiologically of the glutamate-GABA duo in that the first member of the pair is excitatory and the second is inhibitory. Since very little is known about either cysteic acid or taurine, their possible function is still unclear. The function of taurine in liver in conjugating with bile acids to form bile salts lends some support for the hypothesis that it has an analogous role in brain in association with cholic acid derived from cholesterol metabolism.

Isethionate (hydroxyethane sulfonic acid) is formed from taurine by oxidative deamination. Both compounds have been shown to depress drug-induced cardiac excitability; the effects of taurine are considered attributable to its conversion to isethionate. This anion has no known function in mammalian nervous tissue; in some invertebrates it serves as a principal organic anion.

A rather puzzling situation exists with respect to urea in the brain. Arginosuccinate synthetase, the arginosuccinate-splitting enzyme, and arginase have been found in the brain. However, attempts to find carbamyl phosphate synthetase and ornithine transcarbamylase have been negative. It is conceivable that citrulline is not formed from ornithine in brain but is transported there, giving rise to a modified urea cycle that is in point of fact acyclic. The indication in Figure 3-1 that a change in the level of argino-

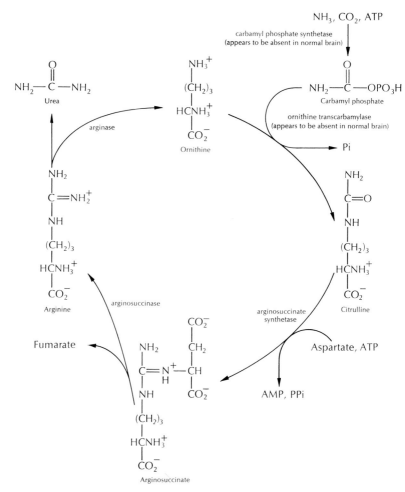

FIGURE 3-2. Urea synthesis.

succinate in the brain is related to a behavioral change stems from findings in a rare genetic disease called arginosuccinic aciduria. In this disease, characterized by a severe mental deficiency and convulsions, large amounts of arginosuccinic acid are excreted in the urine; a high concentration of the compound is also found in the cerebrospinal fluid. Since urinary urea formation is within normal range, it is thought that the genetic block is not in the liver but may well be localized in the brain. The urea cycle is depicted in Figure 3-2.

Finally, to complete the outline in Figure 3-1, we turn to the three essential aromatic amino acids, phenylalanine, tryptophan, and histidine. It is interesting to look at them as a group since (a) they all are associated with inborn errors of metabolism that produce mental retardation and (b) they all give rise to neuroactive amines. In the case of tyrosine (derived from phenylalanine in the liver) and tryptophan, the metabolic pathways are strikingly similar since decarboxylation produces pressor agents (tyramine, tryptamine), whereas oxidation prior to decarboxylation yields presumptive neurotransmitters (dopamine, norepinephrine, epinephrine and serotonin). With histidine, decarboxylation also gives rise to a vaso-active substance (histamine). Although from a structural standpoint it is likely that histidine is converted to ergothioneine, the biosynthesis of this betaine derivative of thiolhistidine has yet to be demonstrated. The excitatory activity of ergothioneine (the "cerebellar factor") on the cerebellum as well as the activity of the neurotransmitters derived from the other aromatic amino acids will be discussed in later chapters.

In this chapter on the biochemistry of the central nervous system no attempt has been made to discuss the two dozen or more genetic abnormalities that are associated with mental retardation; those that are noted are mentioned only because they were associated with compounds that were discussed for other reasons. Aberrant amino acid, carbohydrate, and lipid metabolism may all produce mental deficiencies. Rather than illuminating a specific reaction that is vital to normal mental development, these genetic blocks dramatically point out the necessity of totally integrated metabolism. Table 3-2 lists some genetic abnormalities that are associated with cerebral impairment.

No discussion of nucleic acids and proteins has been presented in this chapter since (a) the synthetic and catabolic pathways of these macromolecules in brain do not appear to be basically different from those in other tissues so that they do not fit into the scheme as shown in Figure 3-1 and (b) their relationship to memory and learning procedures is discussed in Chapter 9. This omission is not meant to imply that proteins of brain are

TABLE 3.2. Hereditary Diseases Associated with Cerebral Impairment

Disorder	Defect
(A) Amino Acid Metabolism	
arginosuccinic aciduria	arginosuccinase
citrullinemia	arginosuccinic acid synthetase
cystathionuria	cystathionine cleaving enzyme
Hartnup disease	trytophan transport
histidinemia	histidase
homocystinuria	cystathionine synthetase
hydroxyprolinemia	hydroxyproline oxidase
hyperammonemia	ornithine transcarbamylase
hyperprolinemia	proline oxidase
maple syrup urine disease	valine, leucine, and isoleucine decarboxylation
phenylketonuria	phenylalanine hydroxylase
(B) Lipid Metabolism	
abetalipoproteinemia (acanthocytosis)	β-lipoproteins
cerebrotendonous xanthomatosis	cholesterol
Gaucher's disease	cerebrosides
juvenile amaurotic idiocy	gangliosides (?)
Krabbe's globoid dystrophy	cerebrosides
Kuf's disease	gangliosides (?)

identical with extraneural proteins. Several soluble proteins have been isolated which immunologically represent brain-specific protein. To date, however, no function has been ascribed to these proteins.

The attempt in this chapter has been to explain the functional uniqueness of brain in terms of biochemistry. To this end we can point to a variety of substrates and reactions that appear to distinguish and characterize nervous tissue, but in reality we have still failed to explain the uniqueness of brain. We still cannot define the particular specialization of the brain on the basis of our current biochemical knowledge. Neither, of course, can we explain biochemically the function of other specialized organs

TABLE 3.2. *Continued*

Disorder	Defect
metachromatic leukodystrophy	sulfatides
Niemann-Pick disease	gangliosides and sphingomyelins
Refsum's disease	3,7,11,15-tetramethylhexadecanoic acid
Tay-Sachs disease	gangliosides
(C) Carbohydrate Metabolism	
galactosemia	galactose-1-phosphate uridyl transferase
glycogen storage disease (type 2)	α-glucosidase
Hurler's disease	chondroitin sulfuric acid β
Umvericht myoclonus epilepsy	polysaccharides (?)
(D) Miscellaneous	
cretinism	thyroid hormone
Hallevorden-Spaatz disease	iron deposition in basal ganglia
intermittent acute porphyria	δ-aminolevulinic acid
subacute necrotizing encephalomyelopathy	thiamine triphosphate
Lesch-Nyhan syndrome	hypoxanthine-guanine phosphoribosyl transferase
Wilson's disease	ceruloplasmin

such as the kidney. This specialization is morphological. The major biochemical contribution is the synthesis of specific macromolecules: the biochemistry of morphogenesis is really DNA → RNA → protein. Nevertheless the reactions discussed in this chapter coupled with the knowledge of neurotransmitters to be presented may be of fundamental importance in explaining the action of neuropharmacological agents.

Angelucci, L. (1956). Experiments with perfused frog's spinal cord. *Brit. J. Pharmacol. 11*, 161.

Bartolini, A., and G. Pepeu (1967). Investigations into the acetylcholine output from the cerebral cortex of the cat in the presence of hyoscine. *Brit. J. Pharmacol. Chemotherap. 31*, 66.

Birks, R., and F. C. MacIntosh (1961). Acetylcholine metabolism of a sympathetic ganglion. *Can. J. Biochem. Physiol. 39*, 787.

De Robertis, E., G. R. L. Arnaiz, and A. D. De Iraldi (1962). Isolation of synaptic vesicles from nerve endings of the rat brain. *Nature 194*, 794.

Edström, A. (1964). The ribonucleic acid in the Mauthner neuron of the goldfish. *J. Neurochem. 11*, 309.

Eichberg, J., Jr., V. P. Whittaker, and R. M. C. Dawson (1964). Distribution of lipids in subcellular particles of guinea pig brain. *Biochem. J. 92*, 91.

Feldberg, W., and V. J. Lotti (1967). Temperature responses to monoamines and an inhibition of MAO injected into the cerebral ventricles of rats. *Brit. J. Pharmacol. Chemotherap. 31*, 152.

Gaitonde, M. K., S. A. Marchi, and D. Richter (1964). The utilization of glucose in the brain and other organs of the cat. *Proc. Roy. Soc. B. 160*, 124.

Geiger, A. (1958). Correlation of brain metabolism and function by the use of a brain perfusion method *in situ*. *Physiol. Rev. 38*, 1.

Giacobini, E. (1965). Metabolism and function studied in single neurones. *Ann. Ist. Super, Sanita. 1*, 500.

Heller, A., J. A. Harvey, and R. Y. Moore (1962). A demonstration of a fall in brain serotonin following CNS lesions in rat. *Biochem. Pharmacol. 11*, 859.

Hydén, H. (1960). *The Cell* (J. Brachet and A. E. Mirsky, Eds.), Vol. 4, Academic Press, New York.

Jacobsen, J. G., and L. H. Smith, Jr. (1968). Biochemistry and physiology of taurine and taurine derivatives. *Physiol Rev. 48*, 424.

Kety, S., and C. F. Schmidt (1948). The nitrous oxide method for the quantitative determination of cerebral blood flow in man: theory, procedure and normal values. *J. Clin. Invest. 27*, 476.

Lowry, O. H. (1963). The Chemical Study of Single Neurons. The Harvey Lectures, Academic Press, New York.

Lowry, O. H., J. V. Passonneau, D. W. Schulz, and M. K. Rock (1961). The measurement of pyridine nucleotides by enzymatic cycling. *J. Biol. Chem. 236*, 2746.

McIlwain, H., and R. Rodnight (1962). *Practical Neurochemistry*, Little, Brown, Boston.

McIlwain H. (1966). *Biochemistry and the Central Nervous System*, Churchill, London.

McIntosh, J. C., and J. R. Cooper (1965). Studies on the function of *N*-acetyl aspartic acid in brain. *J. Neurochem. 12*, 825.

Matsuura, S., Kawaguchi, M. Ichiki, M. Sorimachi, K. Kataoka, and A. Inouye (1969). Perfusion of frog's spinal cord as a convenient method for neuropharmacological studies. *Europ. J. Pharmacol. 6*, 13.

Mitchell, J. F. (1963). The spontaneous and evoked release of acetylcholine from the cerebral cortex. *J. Physiol.* (Lond.) *165*, 98.

Murray, M. R., (1965). *Cells and tissues in culture* (E. W. Willmer, Ed.), vol. 2, Academic Press, New York.

Norton, W. T., and S. E. Podluso (1970). Neuronal soma and whole neuroglia of rat brain; a new isolation technique. *Science 167*, 1144.

Ratner, S., H. Morell, and E. Carvalho (1960). Enzymes of arginine metabolism in brain. *Arch. Biochem. Biophys. 91*, 280.

Roots, B. I., and P. V. Johnson (1967). Neurons of ox brain nuclei: their isolation and appearance by light and electron microscopy. *J. Ultrastruct. Res. 10*, 350.

Rose, S. P. R., (1965). Preparation of enriched fraction from cerebral cortex containing isolated, metabolically active neuronal cells. *Nature 206*, 621.

Whittaker, V. P., J. A. Michaelson, and R. J. Kirkland (1964). The separation of synaptic vesicles from nerve endings particles (synaptosomes). *Biochem. J. 90*, 293.

4 | Acetylcholine

THE NEUROPHYSIOLOGICAL activity of acetylcholine (ACh) has been known since the turn of the century and its neurotransmitter role since the mid-1920's. With this history it is not surprising that the graduate student or medical student assumes that everything is known about this subject. This chapter makes clear that almost the only thing definitely known in any detail about ACh is its structural formula; we cannot at the present time even state with certainty its conformation in solution.

ASSAY PROCEDURES

ACh may be assayed by its effect on biological test systems or by physico-chemical methods. Bioassay preparations include the frog rectus abdominis, the dorsal muscle of the leech, the guinea pig ileum, the rat (or cat) blood pressure, and the heart of Venus mercenaria. In general bioassays tend to be laborious, subject to interference by naturally occurring substances, and on occasion to behave in a mysterious fashion (for example, the frog rectus abdominis is not as sensitive to ACh in the summer months as in the winter, and it is not unusual to encounter a guinea pig ileum that will not respond to ACh). Nevertheless, bioassays at the present time represent the most sensitive ($<$ 1 ng) and, under properly controlled conditions, the most specific procedure for determining ACh. It is probably true to state that the neurochemically oriented investigator's natural fear and distrust of a bioassay have hampered progress in elucidating biochemical and biophysical aspects of ACh. This statement is supported by a consideration of the recent explosion of information on norepinephrine. This neurotransmitter can also be bioassayed, but it was only after the development of sensitive fluorometric and radiometric procedures for determining components of the adrenergic nervous system that the information explosion occurred.

Until about 1965 physico-chemical methods for determining ACh were so insensitive as to be virtually useless in measuring endogenous levels of ACh. However, since then there have been reports published on enzymatic, fluorometric, and gas chromatographic techniques that in theory approach the sensitivity and specificity of the bioassays. One of the major problems to date of these methods is that interference from tissues precludes measuring very small amounts of endogenously formed compound. The second problem is one of a lack of sensitivity. It is hoped that these barriers will shortly be removed.

SYNTHESIS

Acetylcholine is synthesized in a reaction catalyzed by choline acetyltransferase (choline acetylase):

$$\text{acetyl CoA} + \text{choline} \longrightarrow \text{ACh} + \text{CoA}$$

The reaction may be followed by:

1. Incubating acetyl CoA and choline and measuring ACh production by one of the methods mentioned above. An anticholinesterase is usually added to inhibit hydrolysis of the ACh that is formed. Rather than adding acetyl CoA, a number of investigators generate this compound with acetyl phosphate, phosphotransacetylase, and CoA, or alternatively, acetate, ATP, CoA, and acetate thiokinase (acetate activating enzyme, acetyl CoA synthetase).

2. Incubating acetyl-^{14}C-CoA and choline and measuring radioactive ACh after its isolation either by precipitation as an insoluble salt such as the Reineckate or by ion exchange chromatography.

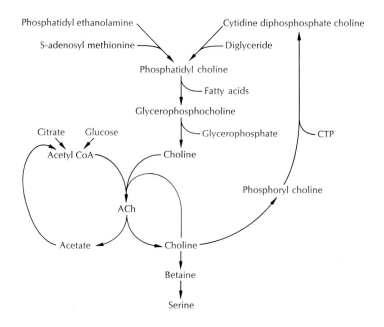

FIGURE 4-1. Acetylcholine metabolism.

Before entering into a discussion of choline acetylase, we should take note of Figure 4-1, which depicts the possible sources of acetyl CoA and choline. In theory, the acetyl CoA for ACh synthesis may arise from glucose, through glycolysis and the pyruvate oxidase system; from citrate, either by a reversal of the condensing enzyme (citrate synthetase) or by the citrate cleavage enzyme; or from acetate through acetatethiokinase. In brain slices, homogenates, acetone powder extracts, and preparations of nerve ending particles, glucose or citrate proved to be the best sources for ACh synthesis, with acetate rarely showing any activity. However, these systems are all *in vitro* and do not necessarily reflect the situation *in vivo*. The only system attempted to date which more nearly represents a physiological condition is that of Fitzgerald. This investigator utilized the ACh-synthesizing capacity of the corneal epithelium (see below) and injected trace amounts of labeled precursors into the anterior chamber of rabbit eyes. Subsequently the corneal epithelium was removed and the radioactive ACh was isolated and determined. In this study it was found that acetate was incorporated into ACh almost ten times more efficiently than glucose, pyruvate, or citrate.

The disposition of choline is still not clear. It may be directly reutilized following the hydrolysis of ACh, or because of transport difficulties (it crosses membranes by an active transport process) it may be initially phosphorylated and then undergo a series of reactions leading to phosphatidyl choline and subsequently ACh. Another possibility, as outlined in Figure 4-1, is that phosphatidyl choline is derived from phosphatidyl ethanolamine, although the turnover of this phospholipid in stimulated nervous tissue is slow. At the present time there is not enough information available to determine what proportion of choline comes from each possible source. From experiments on the superior cervical ganglion both in Feldberg's and in MacIntosh's laboratory (see below) and from the studies of Fitzgerald noted above, it appears that choline is rate-limiting in the synthesis of ACh.

With respect to the cellular localization of choline acetyltransferase, the highest activity is found in the caudate nucleus, retina, corneal epithelium, and central spinal roots (3000 to 4000 μg ACh synthesized/g/hr). In contrast dorsal spinal roots contain only trace amounts of the enzyme, as does the cerebellum.

Intracellularly, after differential centrifugation in a sucrose medium, choline acetyltransferase is found in mammalian brain predominantly in the crude mitochondrial fraction. This fraction contains mitochondria, nerve ending particles (synaptosomes) with enclosed synaptic vesicles, and membrane fragments. When this fraction is subjected to sucrose density gradient centrifugation, the bulk of the choline acetyltransferase is found to be associated with nerve ending particles. When these synaptosomes are ruptured by hypo-osmotic shock, synaptosomal cytoplasm can be separated from synaptic vesicles. In a solution of low ionic strength the choline acetyltransferase is adsorbed to the vesicles, but in the presence of salts at physiological concentration the enzyme is solubilized and remains in the cytoplasm. *In vivo* the enzyme is most likely present in the cytoplasm of the nerve ending particle and not in vesicles.

A cell-free system of choline acetyltransferase was first described by Nachmansohn and Machado in 1943. Since that time the enzyme from squid head ganglia, human placenta, and brain has been partially purified and some of its characteristics have been defined. As partially purified from rat brain, choline acetyltransferase has a molecular weight of about 65,000, with an apparent Michaelis constant (Km) for choline of 4.5×10^{-4} M and for acetyl CoA of 1.1×10^{-5} M. Currently a controversy exists on the extent of the reversibility of the reaction. The enzyme is activated by salts and is inhibited by sulfhydryl reagents. A variety of studies on the substrate specificity of the enzyme indicates that various acyl derivatives both of CoA and of ethanolamine can be utilized by the enzyme. The major gap in our knowledge of choline acetyltransferase is that as yet we do not know of any useful (i.e. potent and specific) direct inhibitor of the enzyme. Hemicholinium inhibits the synthesis of ACh, but indirectly, by preventing the transport of choline across the cell membrane.

HYDROLYSIS

The splitting of ACh into choline and acetic acid may be followed:

1. gasometrically by using a bicarbonate buffer and measuring the evolution of CO_2;
2. by a change in pH recorded either potentiometrically or by a color change in an indicator;
3. by using acetylthiocholine as substrate and measuring the formation of thiocholine colorimetrically with dithiobisnitrobenzoate;
4. by measuring the amount of ACh remaining after incubation.

Everybody agrees that ACh is hydrolyzed by cholinesterases but nobody is sure just how many cholinesterases exist in the body. All cholinesterases will hydrolyze not only ACh but other esters. Conversely, hydrolytic enzymes such as arylesterases, trypsin, and chymotrypsin will not hydrolyze choline esters. The problem in deciding the number of cholinesterases that exist is that different species and organs sometimes exhibit maximal activity with different substrates. For our purposes we will divide the enzymes into two rigidly defined classes: acetylcholinesterase (also called "true" or specific cholinesterase) and butyrocholinesterase (also called "pseudo" or nonspecific cholinesterase; the term "propiono-cholinesterase" is sometimes used since in some tissues propionyl-choline is hydrolyzed more rapidly than butyrylcholine). When distinguishing between the two types of cholinesterases at least two criteria should be used because of the aforementioned species or organ variation.

The first criterion is the optimum substrate. Acetylcholines-terase hydrolyzes ACh faster than butyrylcholine, propionylcho-line, or tributyrin; the reverse is true with butyrocholinesterase. In addition, acetyl-β-methyl choline (methachol) is only split by acetylcholinesterase. That this criterion for distinguishing be-tween the two esterases is not inviolate and must be used along with other indices is illustrated by the fact that the chicken brain acetylcholinesterase will hydrolyze acetyl-β-methyl choline but will also hydrolyze propionylcholine faster than ACh. Also the bee head enzyme will not hydrolyze either ACh or butyrylcho-line but will split acetyl-β-methyl choline.

A second criterion that is used in differentiating the cholin-esterases is the substrate concentration versus activity relationship. Acetylcholinesterase is inhibited by high concentrations of ACh so that a bell-shaped substrate concentration curve results. This is observed also when butyrylcholine or propionylcholine is used. In contrast, butyrocholinesterase is not inhibited by high subtrate concentrations so that the usual Michaelis-Menten type of sub-strate concentration curve is obtained. The reason for this dif-ference is that in acetylcholinesterase there is at least a two-point attachment of substrate to enzyme whereas with butyrocholines-terase the substrate is attached at only one site.

The type of cholinesterase found in a tissue is often a reflection of the tissue. This fact is used as a discriminating index between cholinesterases. In general, neural tissue contains acetylcholinesterase while nonneural tissue usually contains butyrocholinesterase. However, this is a generalization, and some neural tissue (e.g. autonomic ganglia) contains both esterases as do some extraneural organs, e.g. liver, lung. In the blood, erythrocytes contain only acetylcholinesterase while plasma contains butyrocholinesterase, but plasma has primary substrates varying from species to species. Because of its ubiquity, cholinesterase activity cannot be used as an indicator of a cholinergic system.

A final criterion that may be applied to differentiate between the esterases is their susceptibility to inhibitors. Thus the organophosphorus anticholinesterases such as diisopropyl phosphorofluoridate (DFP) are more potent inhibitors of butyrocholinesterase whereas a compound such as WIN8077 (Ambinonium) is about two thousand times better an inhibitor of acetylcholinesterase.

In discussing the various techniques that are used to classify the cholinesterases, we touched on some aspects of the molecular properties of the enzymes. Since very little work has been done on butyrocholinesterase and since no physiological role for this enzyme (or enzymes) has been demonstrated, we will focus our attention on acetylcholinesterase. In sucrose homogenates of mammalian brain, subjected to differential centrifugation, acetylcholinesterase is found both in the mitochondrial and microsomal fractions. The latter, consisting of endoplasmic reticulum and plasma cell membranes, exhibits a higher specific activity. This localization of the enzyme is supported by electron microscopic and histochemical studies which fix the activity at membranes of all kinds both in the CNS and the peripheral nervous system.

Acetylcholinesterase has been crystallized from *Electrophorus electricus*, is electrophoretically homogeneous (crystalline enzymes are not necessarily pure), and has a molecular weight of 260,000. The preparation can hydrolyze 730 mmoles of ACh/mg protein/hr and is thus among the enzymes having the highest turnover number that is known. With respect to the topography of the enzyme the twin-hatted diagram of the anionic and esteratic sites has been reproduced countless times and need not be presented again here. However, some discussion is in order since this was the first enzyme to be dissected at a molecular level. For this initiation into molecular biology we owe a debt of gratitude to Nachmansohn and his colleagues, particularly Wilson. The active center of acetylcholinesterase has two main sub-sites. The first is an anionic site which attracts the positive charge in ACh and the second, about 5Å distant, is an esteratic site which binds the carbonyl carbon atom of ACh. Current information suggests that the anionic site contains at least one carboxyl group, possibly from glutamate, and the esteratic site involves a histidine residue adjacent to serine. The over-all reaction is written as follows:

$$E + ACh \longrightarrow E \cdot ACh \overset{H_2O}{\longrightarrow} E \cdot Acetyl \longrightarrow E + acetic\ acid$$
$$choline$$

Information on the architecture of the active center has been derived not only from kinetic studies using model compounds but from a group of inhibitors known as the anticholinesterases. (The pharmacology of these agents will be discussed in the last section of the chapter.) The anticholinesterases are classified as reversible and irreversible inhibitors of the enzyme. Like ACh, both types of inhibitor acylate the enzyme at the esteratic site. However, in contrast to ACh or to a reversible inhibitor such as physostigmine, the irreversible inhibitors, which are organo-phosphorus compounds, irreversibly phosphorylate the esteratic site. This phosphorylation has been shown to occur on the hydroxyl group of serine when DFP was incubated with purified acetylcholinesterase. It is interesting to note that when trypsin or chymotrypsin is treated with DFP it is also the serine hydroxyl in these proteins that is phosphorylated. Since in solution serine does not react with DFP it has been suggested that in peptide linkage serine (a) is in an oxazoline ring structure which is then susceptible to phosphorylation or (b) that amino acids, such as histidine, which surround serine promote high reactivity in the serine hydroxyl. Although the organo-phosphorus agents (referred to as nerve gases though they are actually oils) are classed as irreversible anticholinesterases, there is a slow detachment of the compounds from the enzyme. Wilson observed that hydroxylamine speeded up this dissociation and regenerated active enzyme. He then set about designing a nucleophilic agent with a spatial structure that would fit the active center of acetylcholinesterase, and did in fact produce a compound which is very active in displacing the inhibitor. This is 2-pyridine aldoxime methiodide (PAM), which has been used with moderate success in treating poisoning from organophosphorus compounds used as insecticides. PAM, with its quaternary ammonium group, does not penetrate the blood-brain barrier well enough to overcome central actions of the anticholinesterase. For this reason atropine is usually used as an antidote along with PAM. It will be recalled that atropine blocks the effect of ACh at neuroeffector sites and has nothing to do with acetylcholinesterase.

The Genesis of the Cholinergic Triad in Neurons

It has already been pointed out that choline acetyltransferase is found in the cytoplasm of nerve ending particles, that acetylcholinesterase is associated with cell membranes of all kinds (synaptosomal, axonal, and glial), and that ACh is localized to some extent in synaptic vesicles. It is now pertinent to inquire how these three components of the cholinergic system arrived at their respective residences.

The phenomenon of axoplasmic flow has been described in Chapter 2. This is the process by which material synthesized in the cell body moves down the axons of the peripheral nerves either consonant with the rate of outgrowth of axons or by an independent mechanism as yet not understood. In the case of choline acetyltransferase a variety of investigators have by ligation and sectioning of peripheral nerves shown that this enzyme originates in the perikaryon and travels down to the nerve terminal. With acetylcholinesterase the situation is still not clear. Again, by sectioning experiments and by the use of irreversible anticholinesterases, it has been demonstrated that the enzyme can be formed in the cell body and then move down an axon, possibly attached to neurotubules as a carrier. On the other hand, local synthesis of the enzyme in axons has also been demonstrated. The latter results are slightly tainted by Schwann cell contamination of the neuronal preparation so that it cannot be stated with certainty that the enzyme is synthesized by neuronal elements alone. Nevertheless, regardless of the possible contribution of satellite cells to axonal synthesis of acetylcholinesterase, it is clear that the enzyme does not necessarily have to originate in the cell body. It should be kept in mind that these studies, both with choline acetyltransferase and acetylcholinesterase, were done in peripheral nerves. In fact as we explore the problem of ACh it will be apparent that for obvious technical reasons much of our information comes from experiments on the peripheral nervous system. The question is how applicable are the results of these investigations to the cholinergic neurons in the central nervous system? In the case of choline acetyltransferase and acetylcholinesterase we do not know if translocations of the enzymes occur in the CNS.

ACh is localized to a large extent in nerve endings and in synaptic vesicles of brain. To our knowledge no one has isolated vesicles from peripheral nerves, so that inferences about a relationship between the quantal release of ACh at neuromuscular junctions and release of ACh from synaptic vesicles in this region have not received experimental support. As discussed earlier, in the brain the synaptic vesicles within nerve ending particles (synaptosomes) tend to cluster at the membrane that is in apposition to the synaptic cleft. How synaptic vesicles are formed and why they cluster at this location are not understood (cf. Chapter 2).

UPTAKE, STORAGE, AND RELEASE OF ACh

Superior Cervical Ganglion

To date the only major and thorough study of ACh turn-over in nervous tissue has been done by MacIntosh and his colleagues using the superior cervical ganglion of the cat. By using one ganglion to assay the resting level of ACh and by perfusing the contralateral organ these investigators have determined the amount of transmitter synthesized and released under a variety of experimental conditions which includes electrical stimulation, the addition of an anticholinesterase to the perfusion fluid, and a perfusion medium of varying ionic composition. Their results may be summarized as follows:

a. During stimulation, ACh turns over at a rate of 8 to 10 per cent of its resting content every minute, i.e. about 24 to 30 ng/min. At rest the turnover rate is about 0.5 ng/min. Since there is no change in the ACh content of the ganglion during stimulation at physiological frequencies it is evident that electrical stimulation not only releases the transmitter but also stimulates its synthesis.

b. Choline is the rate-limiting factor in the synthesis of ACh.

c. In the perfused ganglion, Na^+ is necessary for optimum synthesis and storage, and Ca^{++} is necessary for the release of the neurotransmitter.

d. Newly synthesized ACh appears to be more readily released on nerve stimulation than depot or stored ACh.

e. About half of the choline produced by cholinesterase activity is reutilized to make new ACh.

f. At least three separate stores of ACh in the ganglion are inferred from these studies: "surplus" ACh, considered to be intracellular, which accumulates only in an eserine-treated ganglion and which is not releasable by nerve stimulation; "depot" ACh, which is released by nerve impulses and accounts for about 85 per cent of the original store; and "stationary" ACh, which constitutes the remaining 15 per cent that is nonreleasable.

As stated above, this work on the superior cervical ganglion represents the most complete information on the turnover of ACh in the nervous system.

Brain Slices, Nerve Ending Particles, and Synaptic Vesicles

About thirty years ago Mann, Tennenbaum, and Quastel demonstrated the synthesis and release of ACh in cerebral cortical slices. In the succeeding thirty years these observations have been repeatedly confirmed but only moderately extended. The major finding of interest in all these studies is that in the usual incubation medium the level of ACh in the slices reaches a limit and cannot be raised. In a high K^+ medium the total ACh is increased substantially because much of it leaks into the medium from the slices. These experiments suggest that the intracellular concentration of the neurotransmitter regulates its rate of synthesis. This concept of a negative feedback mechanism is supported by the findings that the administration of drugs such as morphine, oxotremorine, or anticholinesterases only succeed in, at the most, a doubling of the original level of ACh in the brain. Regardless of the dose of the drug, no higher level can be obtained.

The techniques of Whittaker and of De Robertis in isolating nerve ending particles with enclosed synaptic vesicles from brain have provided some new though still inconclusive data on ACh. The drawback of this technique because of the inhomogeneity of the brain has already been mentioned in Chapter 3. For the following reasons current findings tend to discourage the view that synaptic vesicles are the immediate source of ACh which is released on nerve stimulation:

1. Choline acetyltransferase is localized in the cytoplasm of nerve ending particles and not in synaptic vesicles, as originally believed. Thus ACh has to be transported into the vesicles. The demonstration of this transport is presently a matter of debate in the literature.

2. Isolated vesicles contain only 5 to 50 per cent of the total ACh in nerve endings.

3. As deduced from protein turnover studies of vesicle membranes, the half-life of synaptic vesicles is calculated to be about nineteen days.

4. Studies on the superior cervical ganglion and on the phrenic nerve-diaphragm preparation suggest that the ACh which is released with nerve impulses comes from recently synthesized transmitter ACh and not from vesicle-bound ACh.

5. Procedures that alter ACh synthesis and release do not appear to noticeably affect the number, size, or location of vesicles.

It is, of course, possible to argue against every one of the points above and to uphold the vesicle hypothesis which fits in so nicely with the quantal release of ACh as described in Katz's laboratory. Nevertheless, the concept that vesicles are a store of ACh rather than a primary physiological source is more in line with current information.

ACTION OF ACh

In addition to being a neurotransmitter at certain synapses ACh also has an action on membranes that is still not understood with respect to its physiological importance. The neurotransmitter function in terms of sites can be discussed under the headings "proven," "likely," and "possible."

Transmitter

Virtually all the criteria discussed in Chapter 2 for identifying a neurotransmitter are fulfilled by ACh at the neuromuscular junction, in autonomic ganglia, and at postganglionic parasympathetic nerve endings. In addition, in the CNS the motoneuron collaterals to the Renshaw cells have been shown to be cholinergic. Although technically difficult to establish conclusively, it is *likely* that other synapses in the central nervous system are also cholinergic. With the technique of iontophoresis the following sites have been shown to be affected by ACh: caudate nucleus, ventral basal thalamus, lateral geniculate body, the supraoptic nucleus and posteromedial parts of the thalamus, cochlear nucleus, brain stem, and pyramidal cells of the cortex. In support of cholinergic junctions in the central nervous system may be offered the observation of the marked central effects of the anticholinesterases which can penetrate the blood-brain barrier, and of cholinolytic agents such as atropine. With respect to a *possible* neurotransmitter function of ACh there are a few bits of information that suggest that ACh may participate in pain reception. Thus the findings that nettles (*Urtica urens*) contain ACh and histamine, that high concentrations of ACh injected into the brachial artery of humans have been shown to result in intense pain, and that ACh applied to a blister produced a brief but severe pain, all indicate a relationship between ACh and pain. Further, when hemicholinium is instilled in a rabbit eye, the animal loses its corneal reflex concurrently as the ACh content of the corneal epithelium falls and the reflex returns when the ACh level rises to normal values. In addition, local denervation of the rabbit cornea results in a loss of 94 per cent of the ACh content of the tissue ten days after denervation. It should be noted that bradykinin and substance P produce painful reactions when applied at much lower concentrations than is necessary with ACh. That ACh may act as a sensory transmitter in thermal receptors, taste fiber endings, and chemoreceptors has also been suggested, based on the excitatory activity of the compound on these sensory nerve endings.

Membrane Effects

A variety of actions of ACh that may be viewed as membrane effects rather than neurotransmitter activity has been described and is listed below:

1. Stimulation of incorporation of inorganic phosphate into phospholipids: A number of investigators have shown that

ACh at a concentration of about 10^{-4} M will stimulate the incorporation of $^{32}P_i$ into phospholipids, particularly phosphatidyl inositol, and phosphatidic acid. This stimulation has been demonstrated not only in salt gland, sympathetic ganglia, and brain slices but also in brain homogenates. The mechanism of this stimulation has not been rigorously proven but the current evidence suggests that ACh is stimulating the hydrolysis of phosphoinositides in synaptosomes to form membrane-bound diglyceride. It is assumed that the membrane-bound diglyceride is rate limiting in the synthesis of both phosphatidic acid and phosphoinositides.

2. Release of thiamine: Itokawa and Cooper have shown that ACh, as well as a variety of neuroactive drugs, will release thiamine from perfused nerve preparations. This releasing effect can also be demonstrated with membrane preparations from brain, spinal cord, and sciatic nerve, although with this subcellular fraction higher concentrations of ACh are necessary (10^{-4} M in contrast to 10^{-6} M with intact preparations).

3. Release of catecholamines: It has been known for many years that ACh releases catecholamines from chromaffin cells.

4. Conduction: That ACh is involved in the conduction process in axons has been espoused by Nachmansohn for over a quarter of a century. Both his theory and a detailed indictment of it by Koelle can be appraised in the references given at the end of this chapter. Although the evidence against the participation of ACh in conduction is overwhelming, nevertheless no satisfactory explanation has yet been given for the ability of ACh (albeit in high concentrations) to depolarize an axon.

5. Non-nervous tissue: Ciliary movement in the gill plates of *Mytilus edulis* has been observed to be under the control of ACh. Ciliary activity is increased by eserine and inhibited by atropine and *d*-tubocurarine. Ciliary motility of

respiratory and esophageal tracts in mammals also appears to be controlled by ACh.

The depolarizing effect of ACh on intestinal smooth muscle has been shown to be independent of nervous intervention: this action is a direct one on smooth muscle fibers. Similarly, the hyperpolarizing action of ACh on atrial muscle in the absence of nervous control has been demonstrated.

These situations describe an activity of ACh that is independent of innervation. There is also a variety of tissues and organisms, such as human placenta, *Lactobacillus plantarum* and *Trypanosoma rhodesience*, and a fungus (*Claviceps purpurea*) in which ACh is found but where nothing is known of its action.

THE CHOLINERGIC RECEPTOR

Every few years someone states that the cholinergic receptor is in fact acetylcholinesterase. That this belief is erroneous may be construed from the following facts:

1. In the isolated electroplax of *Electrophorus electricus* the apparent dissociation constant of the ACh-receptor complex is 5×10^{-6} M, whereas the Michaelis constant (K_m) of acetylcholinesterase in this preparation is 1×10^{-4} M.

2. Incubation of an electroplax with either p-chloromercuribenzoate or dithiothreitol abolishes the response to ACh but has no effect on either the K_m or V_{max} of acetylcholinesterase.

3. No correlation exists between inhibition of acetylcholinesterase by a variety of methylcarbamates and their depolarizing potencies on the electroplax. In addition, acetyl-β-methyl choline, which is specifically hydrolyzed by acetylcholinesterase, does not depolarize the electroplax.

4. Incubation of an intact skeletal muscle with pronase and other proteases abolishes the cholinesterase activity of the end plate but does not affect the response of the muscle to applied ACh.

Having disposed of the cholinesterase theory it is now incumbent upon us to state that in fact the cholinergic receptor most likely has a topography very similar to the active center of acetylcholinesterase, i.e. anionic and esteratic binding sites. This is virtually a truism, merely from a perusal of the charge distribution on the ACh molecule. In addition the bell-shaped curve obtained from a substrate concentration versus activity plot for acetylcholinesterase is also obtained for cholinergic receptor activity; that is, increased concentrations of ACh inhibit both hydrolysis and response at cholinergic junctional tissue.

Two approaches are currently used to characterize the receptor. The first technique uses intact tissue in which a response of the tissue is measured. This approach is open to the criticism that because one is dealing with at least two events, the combination of drug and receptor and the sequential response of muscle contraction, the primary goal of studying drug-receptor interaction cannot be easily realized. Thus, not only may a problem arise of transport of an agonist or antagonist to the receptor protein but, since the coupling of an activated receptor to a tissue response is not known at a molecular level, it is conceivable that an ACh antagonist may be acting at a further point in the chain.

The second approach used to investigate the cholinergic receptor is an attempt to isolate the receptor substance. From studies on the effects of urea, heat, sulfhydryl-reacting reagents, and proteolytic enzymes, it has been adduced that receptors are proteins (but not enzymes since covalent bonds are not made or broken in the initiation of a response). To this end a number of investigators have isolated proteins which they at one time thought were the cholinergic receptor. Further experimentation has led them to the more modest statement that they have isolated macromolecules which bind drugs. In point of fact it can be argued that it is virtually impossible to isolate and identify a pure receptor since (a) receptors must be in membrane structures. In the isolation, solubilization, and purification of a particulate protein (probably a lipoprotein) one automatically changes its conformation so that binding constants with agonists or antagonists will be altered. (b) The only acceptable proof that a receptor has been isolated will be to put it back in an intact tissue or organ whose receptors have been inactivated and show that the application of a drug will now give the appropriate response. This may be difficult to do.

Drugs That Affect Central Cholinergic Systems

Many of the cholinomimetics, cholinolytics, neuromuscular blocking drugs, and anticholinesterases with which the student is familiar do not affect the central nervous system because of their inability to cross the blood-brain barrier at a significant rate. However, atropine, scopolamine, and DFP (diisopropyl phosphorofluoridate) all penetrate the central nervous system, and their main effects have been studied in some detail.

The systemic injection of atropine and scopolamine leads to a decrease in the ACh content of the brain. This reduction is confined to the cerebral hemispheres. At the same time it has been shown, using the cortical cup technique, that the administration of these drugs either intravenously, intraventricularly, or via the cup resulted in the release of ACh from the exposed cortex into the collecting cup. This releasing effect of ACh by the antimuscarinic agents has also been observed in brain cortical slices. The mechanism by which these agents lower the ACh content of brain and stimulate the release is not known. What is known, however, is that the amnesic effect of atropine and scopolamine does not correlate with the lowered levels of ACh in the brain since the intraventricular injection of hemicholinum, which markedly reduces the ACh concentration in brain, has no effect on maze performance by trained rats.

The administration of oxotremorine and arecoline to rats causes a rise in the ACh content in brain which roughly coincides with the tremor period. This is presumed to be a muscarinic action of these agents since the tremor can be aborted by atropine.

A number of years ago it was observed that the long-term administration of DFP to myasthenics produced nightmares, confusion, and hallucination. Since then a number of studies using different organo-phosphorus anticholinesterases has shown behavioral effects in humans following the acute administration of these agents. Subjects have generally felt agitated, tense, and confused; on psychological tests they showed a slowing of intellectual and motor processes.

There are a variety of phenylglycolate esters (e.g. N-ethyl-2-pyrollidylmethyl-cyclopentylphenylglycolate) which in the peripheral nervous system are classified as anticholinergic drugs. In the CNS these agents appear to be psychotomimetics; depending on the drug and the dose that is given to human subjects, effects range from apprehension to disorientation and delirium. Yohimbine and THA (1,2,3,4-tetrahydro-5-aminoacridine) were shown to antagonize the psychotomimetic effects of the glycolate esters. Interestingly enough, these two compounds are anticholinesterases. Physostigmine is also an antagonist but DFP and Sarin are not; these latter two compounds are hallucinatory by themselves. The conclusion to be drawn from these studies is that the relationship between these drugs and central cholinergic mechanisms is still mysterious.

Changes in the ACh level in brain correlated with behavioral changes in the animal first came into prominence in 1949 when it was shown that during convulsions the ACh level fell, and during sedation the ACh content of the brain rose. These observations have spawned a number of investigations in which an attempt has been made to correlate behavioral changes with the ACh content of brain. A quantity of data has been collected and many papers have been published, but this approach has yet to lead to either an elucidation of the central mechanism of action of a cholinergic drug or the delineation of a cholinergic system in the brain.

Alberquerque, E. X., M. D. Sokoll, B. Sonesson, and S. Thesleff (1968). Studies on the nature of the cholinergic receptor. *European J. Pharmacol. 4*, 40.

Chakrin, L. W., and V. P. Whittaker (1969). The subcellular distribution of (N-Me-³H) acetylcholine synthesized by brain *in vivo. Biochem. J. 113*, 97.

Cholinergic mechanisms (1967), *Ann. N. Y. Acad. Med. 144.*

Collier, B., and F. C. MacIntosh (1969), The source of choline for ACh synthesis in a sympathetic ganglion. *Can. J. Physiol. Pharmacol. 47*, 127.

Ehrenpreis, S., J. N. Fleisch, and T. W. Mittag (1969). Approaches to the molecular nature of pharmacological receptors. *Pharmacol. Rev. 21*, 131.

Fitzgerald, G. C. (1968). Studies on acetylcholine in bovine and rabbit corneal epithelium. Ph.D. Thesis, Yale University.

Hanin, I., and D. J. Jenden (1969). Estimation of choline esters in brain by a new gas chromatographic procedure. *Biochem. Pharmacol. 18*, 837.

Hebb, C., and D. Morris (1969). Identification of acetylcholine and its metabolism. *The Structure and Function of Nervous Tissue*, Academic Press, New York, p. 25.

Itokawa, Y., and J. R. Cooper (1970). Ion movements and thiamine; The release of thiamine from membrane fragments. *Biochem. Biophys. Acta. 196*, 274.

Koelle, G. B. (1961). Cytological distributions and physiological functions of cholinesterases. *Handbuch der experimentellen Pharmakologie*, XV, 268.

Leuzinger, V., M. Goldberg, and E. Carvin (1969). Molecular properties of acetylcholinesterase. *J. Mol. Biol. 40*, 217.

Nachmansohn, D. (1961). Action on axons and role of ACh in axonal conduction. *Handbuch der experimentellen Pharmakologie*, XV, 701.

5 | Catecholamines

THE TERM "catecholamine" refers, generically, to all organic compounds that contain a catechol nucleus (a benzene ring with two adjacent hydroxyl substituents) and an amine group (Fig. 5-1). In practice the term "catecholamine" usually implies dihydroxyphenylethylamine (dopamine, DA) and its metabolic products, norepinephrine (NE) and epinephrine (E).

The great advances in the understanding of the biochemistry, physiology, and pharmacology of norepinephrine and related compounds during the last decade have been made possible mainly through the development of new and sensitive assay techniques.

METHODOLOGY

Bioassay procedures still remain one of the most sensitive methods for the estimation of epinephrine and norepinephrine in tissue extracts or biological fluids and their use is still indicated when dealing with very small amounts of these substances. Table 5-1 gives some of the various bioassay techniques employed for the catecholamines and their relative sensitivities. When the bioassay procedure is coupled with the technique of superfusion, no steps of purification and extraction are necessary and it becomes possible to measure the release and fate of vaso-active hormones directly in the circulation. However, the primary disadvantage of these assay techniques is their relative lack of specificity. The specificity of the bioassay can be increased somewhat by the use

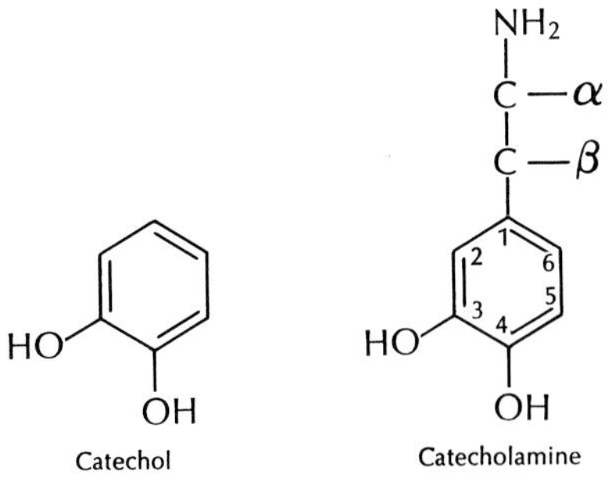

FIGURE 5-1. Catechol and catecholamine structure.

of specific antagonists and the employment of parallel assay systems in which two or more tissues with different sensitivities to the desired agent are employed. This sort of assay system has been employed very elegantly by Vane and his colleagues. Although the bioassay techniques have suitable sensitivity, they have tended to be gradually replaced by chemical methods. This is due mainly to the inherent problems of standardization and specificity.

Fluorometric Assay

The development of sensitive fluorescent techniques for the assay of tissue catecholamines has certainly been a major factor in the rapid advancement of knowledge in this field, in part because the chemical methods do not require the skills of the rapidly vanishing "classical" pharmacologist. Furthermore, fluorescent techniques are also less time-consuming and generally less tedious than the bioassay methods. There are at present two widely used chemical procedures for the estimation of catecholamines after their conversion into fluorescent derivatives: the ethylene diamine condensation method and the trihydroxyindole method. The ethylene diamine condensation method involves the initial oxidation of catecholamines to their intermediate quinone products,

TABLE 5-1. Biological Assay Preparations for Norepinephrine
and Epinephrine

Assay Preparation	Response Measured	Sensitivity Norepineph-rine	Epineph-rine
chick rectal caecum	relaxation	100 ng/ml	1 ng/ml
blood pressure of pithed rat	increase in blood pressure	0.1-1 ng	5-10 ng
rat uterus treated with stilbestrol and contracted with carbachol	relaxation	50 ng/ml	0.5 ng/ml
perfused rabbit ear	increase in perfusion pressure	1-5 ng	1-5 ng
rat stomach strip in presence of serotonin	relaxation	5-20 ng	1-10 ng

which then react with ethylene diamine to form intensely fluorescent products. Since ethylene diamine will condense with many different catechol compounds to give similar fluorescent products, this method is far less specific than the trihydroxyindole reaction, and thus less useful. However, the specificity of this technique can be improved by the employment of suitable separation techniques prior to the analysis. The trihydroxyindole method which involves oxidation and cyclization is more specific and is the procedure commonly used for the assay of catecholamines. The general reaction involved in this assay procedure is illustrated in Figure 5-2. This chemical reaction appears to require the presence of a catechol nucleus, an alkyl amine substituent on the alpha carbon, and a β-hydroxyl group. Although this method is quite sensitive, the detection and estimation of very small amounts of catecholamine (i.e., plasma concentrations) are still quite difficult, due primarily to the instability of the blanks and variable quenching. Udenfriend, in his book on fluorescence

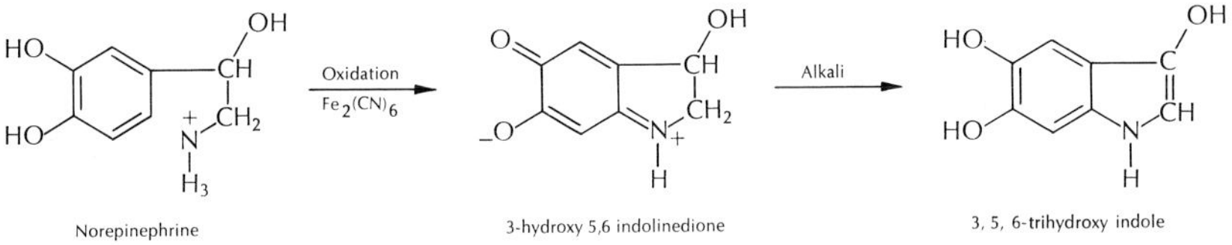

FIGURE 5-2. Trihydroxyindole reaction.

assay, writes, "It is the opinion of this author that in none of the methods currently available has it been possible to establish the identity of apparent norepinephrine in normal plasma."

Gas Chromatography

Gas chromatography is a notable advance in the field of analytical instrumentation, simultaneously providing a suitable means for separation, characterization, and quantitation of the complex organic mixtures encountered in tissue extracts. This technique is just beginning to be used for the identification and quantitation of catecholamines and their metabolites in biological fluids and in tissue extracts. A highly sensitive gas chromatographic technique involves the formation of halogenated catechol derivatives. These derivatives, due to their high electron affinity, make it easy to detect nanogram amounts of material by means of an electron capture detector. In most cases the trifluoroacetyl derivatives have been employed because these compounds have superior chromatographic properties, are readily synthesized, and the unreacted trifluoroacetic anhydride is easily removed by volatilization. Some proven applications include the analysis of 3-methoxy-4-hydroxyphenylglycol in urine, brain and spinal fluid, analysis of 3-methoxy-4-hydroxymandelic acid in urine and the analysis of norepinephrine, normetanephrine, dopamine, and epinephrine in urine and in neuroblastoma and pheochromocytoma tissue. However, this analytical technique has not been utilized to its fullest capacity at the present time, due mainly to the inherent problems of electron capture analysis. Thus, derivative and detector instability as well as frequent contamination of these sensitive detectors presents serious obstacles which must be overcome before this technique will gain wide acceptance.

Radioisotopic Methods

Recently some very sensitive and specific radiochemical assays have been developed for the determination of catecholamine content in biological fluid and tissue. One method is based on the conversion of norepinephrine and epinephrine to their corresponding radioactive derivatives either by incubation with S-adenosyl-L-methionine-methyl-^{14}C and the partially purified enzyme catechol-O-methyl transferase to form O-methyl derivatives or with phenylethanolamine-N-methyl-transferase (commercially available) to form epinephrine. A second method employs tritiated acetic anhydride to produce stable radioactive acetyl derivatives. In both of these methods addition of tracer amounts of ^{3}H- or ^{14}C-labeled catecholamines to the tissue or biological fluid prior to extraction and analysis serves to correct for any losses incurred throughout the procedure. The radioactive derivatives are then subjected to a series of rigorous purification steps prior to analysis. Determination of endogenous levels of catecholamine is then based on the ^{14}C/^{3}H ratios of these purified derivatives. These procedures not only have greater sensitivity than the other methods described but in addition have the decided advantage that the calculation of the amount of amine present is based on a ratio rather than an absolute amount, with the results obtained independent of losses incurred in the purification procedures. In addition, if the radioactivity ratio remains constant through two or more chromatographic procedures, this provides intrinsic evidence of sample purity. This double isotope technique would also be adaptable to gas chromatography, where advantage of the high potential for resolution of related structural compounds can be utilized. This approach is feasible since microgram amounts of unlabeled derivatives can be added to the extracts as carrier, greatly improving the resolution and recovery aspects of this analytic technique.

Histochemical Fluorescence Microscopy and Microspectrofluorometry

In 1955 Eränko, and also Hillarp and Hokfelt, independently observed that fluorescence microscopic examination of adrenal medullary tissue fixed in formaldehyde revealed a bright yellow fluorescence, which they attributed to catecholamines. However, attempts in sympathetically innervated tissue remained unsuccessful for a number of years, probably due to the lower amine concentrations and to the diffusion of the fluorophores into the aqueous fixative. In fact, it was not until 1961 when Falck and his coworkers described the application of freeze drying and treatment of tissue sections with dry formaldehyde vapor that a sufficiently sensitive technique became available for the purpose of demonstrating the very small amounts of catecholamines present in adrenergic nerves. Essentially, this method is based upon the conversion of various ring hydroxylated phenylethylamines, indolealkylamines, and their respective α-amino acids (even histamine) to highly fluorescent derivatives in the presence of relatively dry formaldehyde vapor at 60 to 80° C. This reaction appears to in-

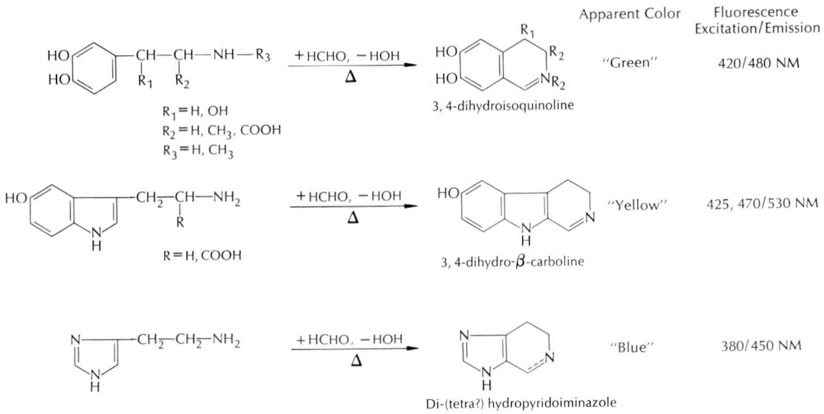

FIGURE 5-3. Formaldehyde condensation products of biogenic monoamines. (Courtesy of Dr. L. S. Van Orden III)

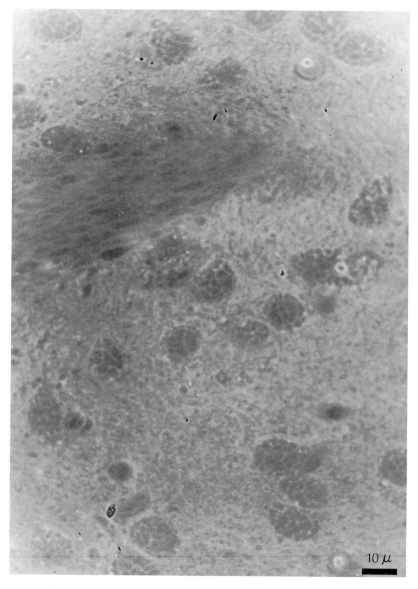

FIGURE 5-4. (A) Normal rat. Transverse section through the caudate nucleus. — equals 10 microns.

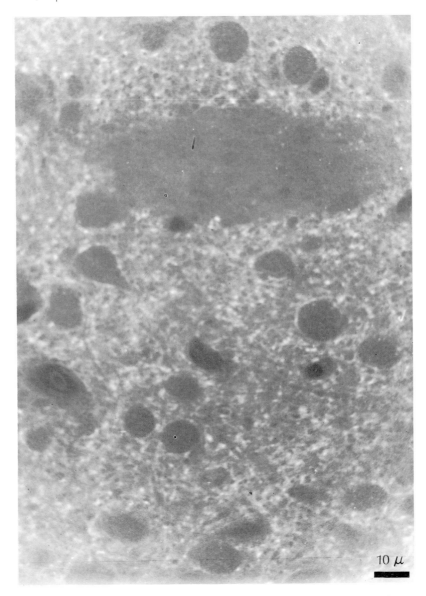

FIGURE 5-4. (B) Rat treated with γ-butyrolactone 750 mg/kg for 90 minutes. Transverse section through the caudate nucleus. — equals 10 microns.

volve the condensation of the amino group with formaldehyde to form a new ring system. The general reaction for phenylethylamines, indolealkylamines, and histamine are illustrated in Figure 5-3. Each of these fluorescent condensation products has its own characteristic fluorescent excitation and emission maximum and therefore one can be distinguished from another spectrally.

One of the main disadvantages of this histochemical technique is that it has been virtually impossible to distinguish spectrally between the reaction products of dihydroxyphenylalanine, dopamine, norepinephrine, and epinephrine since they all form fluorophores with identical fluorescent properties. However, a recent report has indicated that epinephrine and other secondary catecholamines can be distinguished from primary catecholamines because their reaction with formaldehyde requires a much longer time for completion.

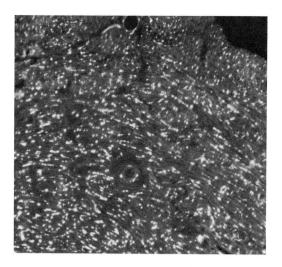

FIGURE 5-5. Fluorescence micrograph, of rat vas deferens. Falck-Hillarp formaldehyde vapor treatment of freeze-dried vas deferens. Magnification approximately 500 x. (Supplied through the courtesy of Dr. L. S. Van Orden, III.)

Recently, Aghajanian and Roth have developed a specific pharmacological method for visualization of brain dopamine. This method is based on the observation that γ-butyrolactone produces a marked increase in brain dopamine without causing a significant increase in brain norepinephrine or serotonin and thus allows a visualization of otherwise largely undetectable fine varicose fluorescent dopamine-containing fibers. Figure 5-4 illustrates a section from the caudate nucleus of a control rat and of a rat treated with γ-butyrolactone. The fluorescence in the dopamine-containing neurons can be seen in the treated rat in Figure 5-4. Currently,

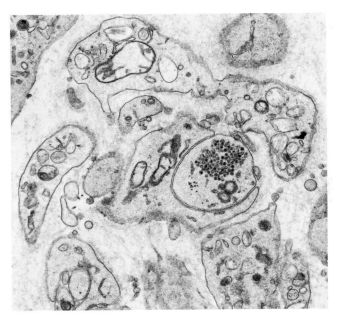

FIGURE 5-6. Electron micrograph of rat iris. Potassium permanganate fixation. A cross section of an adrenergic nerve terminal or "varicosity" containing many synaptic vesicles, most with electron-opaque core (i.e. granular vesicles). Magnification approximately 18,000 x. (Supplied through the courtesy of Dr. L. S. Van Orden, Ill.)

however, most investigators employ complex pharmacological methods to distinguish between norepinephrine and dopamine. Another limitation of the fluorescence method often overlooked by many investigators is that fluorescence intensity of the catecholamine fluorophores is not proportional to amine concentration over a very wide range and therefore the usefulness of this technique remains on a qualitative rather than a quantitative level. In fact, Van Orden *et al.* have demonstrated that the fluorescence histochemical method does not detect granular norepinephrine to the same extent as extragranular norepinephrine.

One must, however, be careful not to underestimate the significance of the contribution of fluorescence histochemistry to the study of catecholamines. The localization of catecholamines and their precursors within morphologically recognizable microscopic structures has provided a great advantage to those investigators interested in studying and understanding adrenergic mechanisms (Fig. 5-5). This technique has also been employed in conjunction with electron microscopy quite successfully in the peripheral nervous system where it is possible to obtain a correlation between morphological changes (fluorescence intensity, content of granular vesicles) and monoamine content (Fig. 5-6). Obviously, the lack of such a suitable histochemical technique for the visualization of acetylcholine has proven a serious handicap for those interested in cholinergic mechanisms.

The fluorescence histochemical technique applied to the central nervous system has revealed catecholaminergic neuronal pathways and cell bodies which were previously unrecognized by the conventional methods of neuroanatomy and has made possible an extensive mapping of monoaminergic pathways in brain. Figure 5-7 represents a schematic diagram of the distribution of some of these monoaminergic pathways found in the central nervous system. The anterograde and retrograde changes occurring after nerve sectioning have made it possible to map the ascending and descending monoamine systems within the central nervous system. The concurrent employment of this technique with administration of new potent inhibitors of monoamine biosynthesis (see

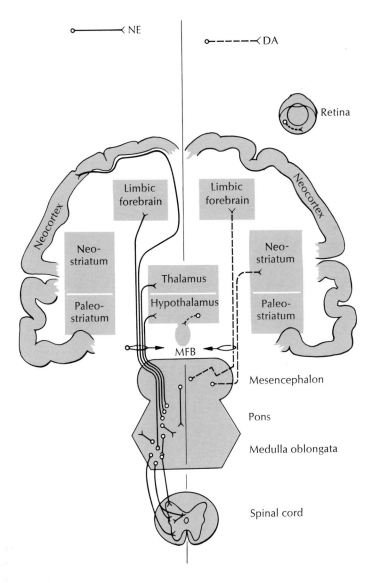

FIGURE 5-7. Central noradrenergic and dopaminergic tracts (modified after Anden *et al.*, *Acta physiol. scand.* 67, 313, 1966).

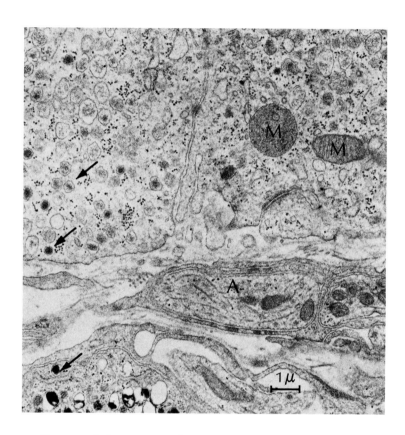

FIGURE 5-8. Low-power electron micrograph of adrenal medulla showing chromaffin granules of varying electron opacity (arrows). Mitochondria can be seen within the chromaffin cell at the top (M), as well as in the unmyelinated axons lying between the chromaffin cells in the middle of the field (A). Note the variability in the electron-opacity of the chromaffin granules between the two cells at the top and the cell at the bottom. This difference in electron density is presumably due to the type of catecholamine stored in the granule.

below) has made it possible to evaluate to some extent the effect of various neurotropic drugs on the activity of central monoaminergic neurons.

In the central nervous system it appears that practically the entire monoamine is contained within enlargements of the nerve terminals. These varicosities or nerve terminal regions have been estimated by fluorescence microscopy to contain very high concentrations of catecholamines, approx. 1000 to 10,000 μg/gm. On

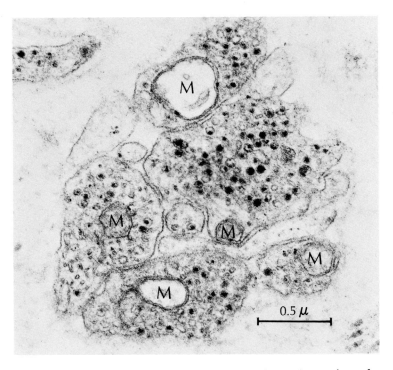

FIGURE 5-9. Sympathetic nerve endings from the perivascular space of the rat pineal. Each nerve terminal exhibits a large number of small granular vesicles, in which electron dense precipitates can be seen. Five mitochondria (M) can be seen within these same nerve terminals. Note the difference in magnification between Figs. 5-8 and 5-9.

the other hand, the monoamine cell bodies and axons have a much lower content (10-100 µg/gm). It is felt by most investigators that these varicosities, due to their relatively high amine content, are the presynaptic structures involved in transmitter storage, release, re-uptake, and synthesis.

Electron Microscopy

In neuropharmacological research, special attention has been devoted to the problem of high resolution cytochemical methods for the identification of synaptic transmitter substances in intact

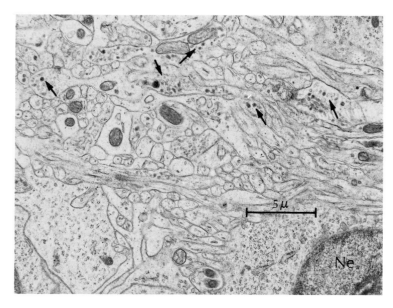

FIGURE 5-10. Low-power electron micrograph from the hypothalamus of a rat showing several axons exhibiting large granular vesicles (arrows). In the nerve terminals exhibiting large granular vesicles, smaller electron-lucent vesicles can be seen, which are of the same size as the small granular vesicles seen in the pineal nerve endings of Fig. 5-9. The nucleus of an ependymal cell can be seen at lower right.

nervous tissue, since this essential criterion must be satisfied in order to identify a substance as the likely transmitter for a particular defined synaptic complex. Thus electron microscopy coupled with the proper cytochemical techniques has provided the investigator in the catecholamine field with a technique for visualization of granular vesicles within the neuron suspected but not proven to contain catecholamines. Figures 5-6 and 5-8 to 11, electron micrographs of rat iris, adrenal medulla, pineal gland, hypothalamus, and cerebellar cortex, illustrate the various types of vesicular structures found in these tissues.

DISTRIBUTION

No matter what our particular specialty in neuropharmacology, we are all ultimately interested in how the agent or agents we wish to study are distributed in the nervous system.

In 1946 von Euler in Sweden and shortly later Holtz in Germany independently identified the presence of norepinephrine in adrenergic nerves. These findings laid the foundation for a new era of research in the field of catecholamines. At that time it was not technically possible to study the content of transmitter in the terminal parts of the adrenergic fiber. Despite this, Euler predicted that norepinephrine was, in fact, highly concentrated in the nerve terminal region from which it was released to act as a neurotransmitter. This prediction was conclusively documented some ten years later with the development of the fluorescence histochemical technique.

A systematic study of extracts of various mammalian nerves by Euler and his colleagues demonstrated that there was a very close correlation between the content of norepinephrine present and the proportion of nonmyelinated to myelinated nerve fibers. Sympathetic ganglia were also found to contain norepinephrine in a concentration similar to that found in the postganglionic fibers. Of all the nerves studied, splenic nerve was found to have the highest content of norepinephrine. This finding is in agreement with histochemical and physiological evidence which indicates that this nerve is made up almost exclusively of small non-myelinated adrenergic fibers. This tissue serves therefore as an excellent model system to study synthesis and storage of the sympathetic neurotransmitter. The correlation between the nor-epinephrine content of a nerve or an organ and its content of adrenergic fibers is now so well established that the occurrence

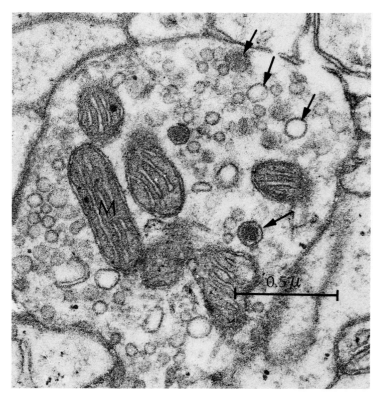

FIGURE 5-11. High-power view of nerve terminal from the cere-bellar cortex exhibiting both small electron-lucent synaptic vesi-cles and large granular vesicles of varying internal electron opacity (arrows). Mitochondria (M) and numerous small elec-tron-lucent synaptic vesicles can also be seen within this nerve terminal.

of NE in a given organ or nerve can, in general, be taken as evidence for the presence of adrenergic fibers provided the presence of chromaffin tissue can be excluded. Table 5-2 illustrates the distribution of norepinephrine in various organs and tissues. Thus, tissues with a high density of sympathetic innervation have a relatively high concentration of sympathetic transmitter, norepinephrine, and vice versa. The rather ubiquitous distribution of norepinephrine in tissue is consistent with the presence of adrenergic vasomotor fibers in almost all peripheral tissue. The absence of norepinephrine in placenta or bone marrow is in agreement with histochemical and physiological evidence, which suggests that these tissues also lack any adrenergic vasomotor innervation.

Shortly after it was established that norepinephrine was the neurotransmitter substance of adrenergic nerves in the peripheral nervous system, norepinephrine was identified by Holtz as a nor-

TABLE 5.2. Tissue Distribution of Norepinephrine
(μg/gm)

Organ	Species			
	Bovine	Cat	Rabbit	Rat
artery	0.2-1.0			
heart	0.48	0.5-1.0	1.4[b]	0.65
liver	0.25	0.005-0.20		0.06
lung	0.05		0.05-0.07[b]	
skeletal muscle	0.04	0.03		
spleen	1.5-3.5	0.8-1.4	0.3-0.5	0.40
splenic nerve	8.5-18.5			
vas deferens	9.3[a]	4.4[a]	6.7[a]	7.9[a]
vein	0.1-0.5		1.0-2.5[b]	

Unless indicated otherwise data taken from table 18—U.S. von Euler, Noradrenaline

[a] W. O. Sjostrand, Acta Physiol. Scand. 65, Suppl. 257, 1965.
[b] R. H. Roth and J. Hughes, unpublished data.

mal constituent of mammalian brain. However, for some years it was believed that the presence of norepinephrine in mammalian brain only reflected vasomotor innervation to the cerebral blood vessels. It was not until 1954 that Vogt demonstrated that norepinephrine was not uniformly distributed in the central nervous system and that this nonuniform distribution did not in any way coincide with the density of blood vessels found in a given brain area. This characteristic regional localization of norepinephrine within mammalian brain suggested that norepinephrine might subserve some specialized function perhaps as a central neurotransmitter. In fact, this observation undoubtedly supplied the impetus for many investigators to pursue actively the functional reasons for the nonuniform presence of this active substance in the central nervous system. The relative distribution of norepinephrine is quite similar in most mammalian species. The highest concentration is usually found in the hypothalamus and other areas of central sympathetic representation. More norepinephrine is generally found in gray matter than in white matter.

Dopamine is also found in the mammalian central nervous system and its distribution differs markedly from that of norepinephrine, suggesting that dopamine is present not only as a precursor of norepinephrine. In fact, it represents more than 50 per cent of the total catecholamine content of the central nervous system of most mammals. The highest levels of dopamine are found in the neostriatum, nucleus accumbens, and tuberculum olfactorium. The presence of abundant dopamine in the basal ganglia has stimulated intensive research on the functional aspects of this compound. There is a growing wealth of evidence which suggests that this agent may have an important role in extrapyramidal function. Some cases of Parkinsonism, a disease characterized by extrapyramidal symptomatology such as rigidity, akinesia, and tremor can be improved by daily administration of large amounts of DOPA (dihydroxyphenylalanine), the immediate precursor of dopamine. All the neurochemical findings with respect to this disease suggest that, generally speaking, there is a decreased ability of the affected brain tissue to form or retain dopamine. Table 5-3

TABLE 5-3. Catecholamine Distribution in the Central Nervous System

Brain Region	Species	Dopamine µg/gm	Norepinephrine µg/gm
whole brain	dog	0.19	0.16
whole brain	rabbit	0.32	0.29
whole brain	rat	0.60	0.49
whole brain	cat	0.28	0.22
medulla oblongata	dog	0.13	0.37
medulla oblongata	rat	—	0.72
mesencephalon	dog	0.10	0.41
cerebellum	rat	—	0.17
cerebellar cortex	dog	0.03	0.06
hypothalamus	rat	0.14	1.29
hypothalamus	dog	—	1.00
hypothalamus	cat	—	1.40
striatum	rat	7.50	0.25
caudate nucleus	rat	6.39	0.27
caudate nucleus	cat	9.90	0.10
caudate nucleus	dog	5.90	0.10
lentiform nucleus	dog	1.63	0.08
cerebral cortex	dog	—	0.05
cerebral cortex	rat	0.01	0.18

Data taken from: L. L. Iversen, *The Uptake and Storage of Noradrenaline in Sympathetic Nerves*, Cambridge Univ. Press. 1967, p. 34.

summarizes the regional brain distribution of norepinephrine and dopamine in various mammalian species.

Epinephrine concentration in the mammalian central nervous system is relatively low, approximately 5 to 17 per cent (by bioassay) of the norepinephrine content. Many investigators have suggested that these estimates are subject to error and have therefore discounted the importance of the occurrence of epinephrine in mammalian brain. However, recently it has been demonstrated that certain brain areas such as the olfactory bulb and olfactory tubercle contain substantial amounts of the enzyme phenylethanolamine-*N*-methyl transferase and therefore are capable of forming epinephrine *in vivo*. At present, the significance of the presence or synthetic capacity for epinephrine in certain brain areas is unknown, but it is conceivable that epinephrine might play some role as a neurohumoral agent in mammalian olfactory structures.

A detailed topographical survey of brain catecholamines at different levels of organization within the central nervous system has helped to give us some sort of basic framework from which to organize and conduct logical experiments concerning the possible function of these amines.

Intraneuronal Localization

With the refinement of physical and chemical techniques it became possible to further localize monoamines both in isolated subcellular particles obtained by differential and density gradient centrifugation and by fluorescence histochemistry and electron microscopy in axonal varicosities. These powerful techniques have provided us with our current concepts concerning the location of amines within the neuron in a structure referred to as synaptic vesicles. The concept of storage of monoamines, however, will be covered in more detail when we consider the life cycle of the catecholamines.

LIFE CYCLE OF THE CATECHOLAMINES

Biosynthesis

Catecholamines are formed in brain, chromaffin cells, sympathetic nerves, and sympathetic ganglia from their amino acid precursor tyrosine by a sequence of enzymatic steps first postulated by Blaschko in 1939 and finally confirmed by Nagatsu in 1964 with the demonstration that an enzyme (tyrosine hydroxylase) was involved in the conversion of L-tyrosine to DOPA. This amino acid precursor, tyrosine, is normally present in the circulation in a concentration of about 5 to 8×10^{-5}M. It is taken up from the bloodstream and concentrated within the brain and presumably also in other sympathetically innervated tissue by an active transport mechanism. Once inside the peripheral neuron tyrosine undergoes a series of chemical transformations resulting in the ultimate formation of norepinephrine or in brain, norepinephrine, dopamine, or epinephrine, depending upon the availability of phenylethanolamine-N-methyl transferase or dopamine β-hydroxylase. This biosynthetic pathway for the formation of catecholamines is illustrated in Figure 5-12. The conversion of tyrosine to norepinephrine and epinephrine was first demonstrated in the adrenal medulla. More recently, the availability of radioactive precursors of high specific activity and chromatographic separation techniques has allowed the confirmation of the above-mentioned pathway to norepinephrine in sympathetic nerves, ganglia, heart, arterial and venous tissue, and brain. In mammals, tyrosine can be derived from dietary phenylalanine by a hydroxylase (phenylalanine hydroxylase) found primarily in liver. Both phenylalanine and tyrosine are normal constituents of mammalian brain, present in a free form in a concentration of about 5×10^{-5}M. However, norepinephrine biosynthesis is usually considered to begin with tyrosine which represents a branch point for many important biosynthetic processes in animal tissues (Fig. 5-13). It should be emphasized that the percentage of tyrosine utilized for catecholamine biosynthesis as opposed to other biochemical pathways is very minimal.

     1. *Tyrosine hydroxylase.* The first enzyme in the biosynthetic pathway, tyrosine hydroxylase, was the last enzyme in this series of reactions to be identified. It was demonstrated by Udenfriend and his colleagues in 1964 and its properties have recently been reviewed. It is present in the adrenal medulla, brain, and in all sympathetically innervated tissue studied to date. However, it has not yet been shown to be a unique constituent of the sympathetic neuron and the adrenal medulla. It does, however, completely disappear from renal, salivary gland, vas deferens, and cardiac tissue upon chronic denervation. The enzyme is stereospecific, requires molecular O_2, Fe^{++}, and a tetrahydropteridine cofactor, and shows a fairly high degree of substrate specificity. Thus, this enzyme, in contrast to tyrosinase, oxidizes only the naturally oc-

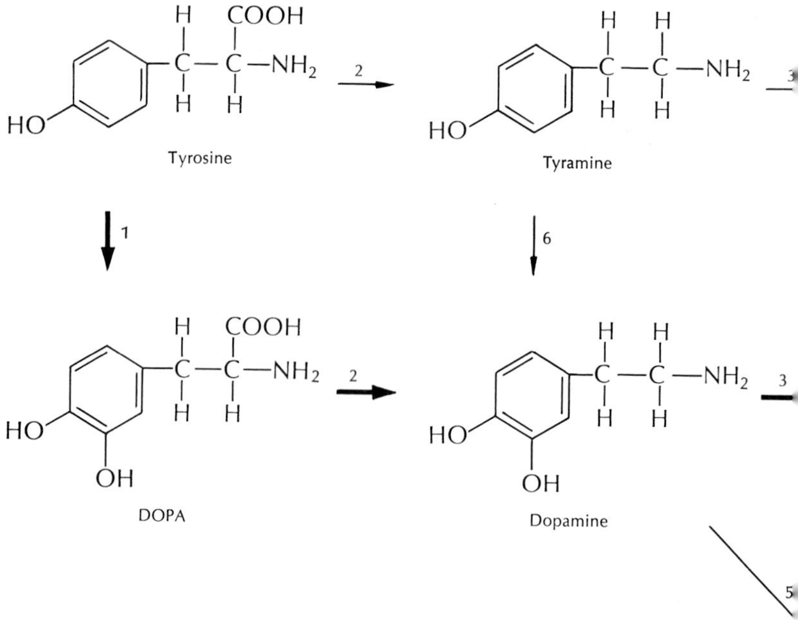

FIGURE 5-12. Primary and alternative pathways in the formation of catecholamines:
1. Tyrosine hydroxylase 2. Aromatic amino acid decarboxylase
3. Dopamine-β-oxidase 4. Phenylethanolamine - N-methyl transferase 5. Non-specific N-methyl transferase in lung.
6. Catechol-forming enzyme.

curring amino acid, L-tyrosine, and to a smaller extent L-phenyl-alanine D-tyrosine, tyramine, or L-tyrptophan will not serve as substrates for the enzyme. However, phenylalanine hydroxylase and tyrosine hydroxylase appear to be distinct enzymes since phenyl-alanine hydroxylase does not hydroxylate tyrosine and is not inhibited by some potent tyrosine hydroxylase inhibitors. It has been suggested, but not proven, that the cofactor for tyrosine hydroxylase may be dihydrobiopterin, the compound demonstrated to be a naturally occurring cofactor for phenylalanine hydroxylase. The majority of experiments suggests that the enzyme is present in the particulate-free fraction of nerve or adrenal medullary homogenate,

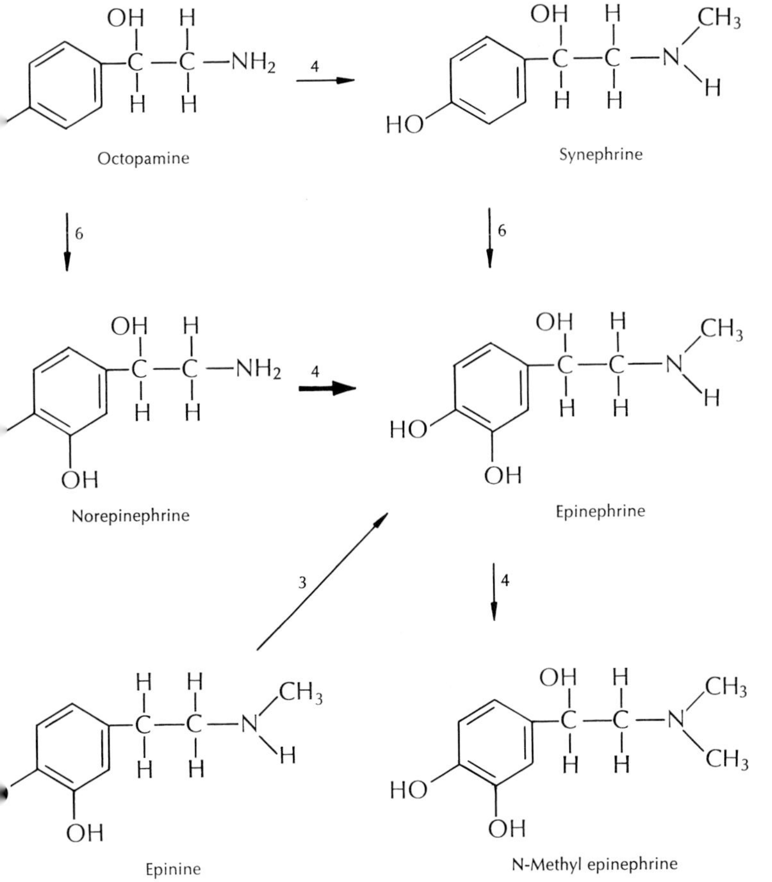

Octopamine → Synephrine

Norepinephrine → Epinephrine

Epinine

N-Methyl epinephrine

although some evidence exists to the contrary. In brain the enzyme is associated with the synaptosome fraction.

The K_m for the enzymatic conversion of tyrosine to DOPA by purified adrenal tyrosine hydroxylase is about $2 \times 10^{-5}M$, and in a preparation of brain synaptosomes about $0.4 \times 10^{-5}M$. Tyrosine hydroxylation appears to be the rate limiting step in the biosynthesis of norepinephrine in the peripheral nervous system and is likely to be the rate limiting step in the formation of norepinephrine and dopamine in the brain as well. In most sympathetically innervated tissues including the brain, the activity of DOPA decarboxylase and that of dopamine-β-oxidase have a

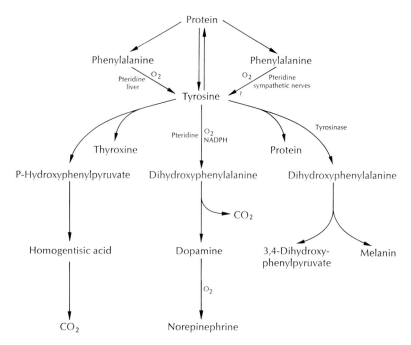

FIGURE 5-13. Metabolism of tyrosine.

magnitude 100 to 1000 times that of tyrosine hydroxylase. This lower activity of tyrosine hydroxylase may be due either to the presence of less enzyme or to a lower turnover number of the enzyme. Since this enzyme has been demonstrated to be the rate limiting step in catecholamine biosynthesis it is logical that pharmacological intervention at this step would cause a reduction of norepinephrine biosynthesis. Many earlier attempts to produce chemical sympathectomy by blockade of the last two steps in the synthesis of norepinephrine have proved largely unsuccessful. On the other hand, studies with inhibitors of tyrosine hydroxylase have proved to be much more successful, producing a marked reduction in endogenous norepinephrine and dopamine in brain and norepinephrine in heart, spleen, and other sympathetically innervated tissues. Effective inhibitors of this enzymatic step can be categorized by four main groups: (1) amino acid analogues; (2) catechol derivatives; (3) tropolones and (4) selective iron chelators. Some effective amino acid analogues include α-methyl-p-tyrosine and its ester, α-methyl-3-iodotyrosine, 3-iodo-tyrosine and α-methyl-5-hydroxytryptophan. In general, α-methyl-amino acids are more potent than the unmethylated analogues, and a marked increase in activity in the case of the tyrosine analogues can also be produced by substituting a halogen at the 3 position of the benzene ring. Most of the agents in this category act as competitive inhibitors of the substrate tyrosine. In this respect α-methyl-5-hydroxytryptophan appears to be unique, since it does not appear to compete with substrate or pteridine cofactor. Its actual mechanism at the present time remains unknown. The potent halogenated tyrosine analogues such as 3-iodotyrosine are about 100 times as active as α-methyl-p-tyrosine *in vitro*, but they are substantially less active *in vivo*. This is probably due to the very rapid deiodination of these compounds to tyrosine or tyrosine analogues which occurs *in vivo*. α-methyl-p-tyrosine and its methyl ester have been the inhibitors most widely used to demonstrate the effects of exercise, stress, and various drugs on the turnover of catecholamines and also to lower norepinephrine formation in patients with pheochromocytoma and malignant hypertension.

A new and rather unique pharmacological agent has been discovered which should be helpful in the study of adrenergic mechanisms. This compound is 6-hydroxydopamine (3, 4, 6-trihydroxyphenylethylamine). When administered intravenously or intraventricularly this compound is rapidly and efficiently taken up into the sympathetic nerve endings. Perhaps because of its selective distribution and concentration as well as its extreme susceptibility to oxidation, this agent appears selectively to destroy sympathetic neurons by causing acute degeneration of adrenergic terminals. In effect this compound produces a "chemical sympathectomy." Thus, when the compound is given intravenously to animals it causes almost total depletion of norepinephrine in sympathetically innervated tissues and also greatly reduces tyrosine hydroxylase activity. The only exception appears to be the adrenal medulla where 6-hydroxydopamine is not effectively taken up and the resultant demands placed on this organ to maintain homeostasis leads to a significant increase in tyrosine hydroxylase activity in this organ. In most aspects, "chemical sympathectomy" produces effects comparable to those produced by surgical denervation or immunosympathectomy. However, this technique has the additional advantage that it may be applied to the central nervous system. Thus, when this agent is given intraventricularly or intracerebrally, it produces an extensive and lasting depletion of brain norepinephrine and a degeneration of central dopamine- and norepinephrine-containing neurons. If it can be shown that this agent acts specifically only to destroy sympathetic neurons, it might well serve as a tool for the evaluation of some of the functional roles ascribed to catecholamines in the central nervous system.

Dihydroxyphenylalanine Decarboxylase

The second enzyme involved in catecholamine biosynthesis is DOPA decarboxylase, which was actually the first catecholamine synthetic enzyme to be discovered. Although originally believed to remove carboxyl groups only from L-DOPA, a study of purified enzyme preparations and specific inhibitors has subsequently demonstrated that this DOPA decarboxylase acts on all naturally occurring aromatic L-amino acids, including histidine, tyrosine, tryptophan, and phenylalanine as well as both DOPA and 5-hydroxytryptophan. Therefore, this enzyme is appropriately referred to as "L-aromatic amino acid decarboxylase." There is no appreciable binding of this enzyme to particles within the cell, since when tissues are disrupted and the resultant homogenates centrifuged at high speeds, the decarboxylase activity remains associated largely with the supernatant fraction. The exception to this is in brain where some of the decarboxylase activity is associated with synaptosomes. However, since synaptosomes are in essence pinched-off nerve endings they would be expected to retain entrapped cytoplasm as well as other intracellular organelles. DOPA-decarboxylase is, relative to other enzymes in the biosynthetic pathway for norepinephrine formation, very active and requires pyridoxal phosphate (vitamin B_6) as a cofactor. The apparent K_m value for this enzyme is $4 \times 10^{-4}M$. The high activity of this enzyme may explain why it has been difficult to detect endogenous DOPA in sympathetically innervated tissue and brain. It is rather ubiquitous in nature, occurring in the cytoplasm of most tissue including the liver, stomach, brain, and kidney in high levels, suggesting that its function in metabolism is not limited solely to catecholamine biosynthesis. Although decarboxylase activity can be reduced by production of vitamin B_6 deficiency in animals, this does not usually result in a reduction of tissue catecholamines although it appears to interfere with the rate of repletion of adrenal catecholamines after insulin depletion. In addition, potent decarboxylase inhibitors also have very little effect on endogenous levels of norepinephrine in tissue.

Dopamine-β-oxidase

Although it has been known for many years that brain, sympathetically innervated tissue, sympathetic ganglia, and adrenal medulla could transform dopamine into norepinephrine, it was not until 1960 that the enzyme responsible for this conversion was isolated from the adrenal medulla. This enzyme requires molecular oxygen and ascorbate and has a K_m of about 5×10^{-3}M. Dicarboxylic acids such as fumaric acid are not absolute requirements, but they stimulate the reaction. Dopamine-β-hydroxylase is a Cu^{++}-containing protein, with about two moles of cupric ion/ mole of enzyme. It appears to be associated with the particulate fraction from heart, brain, sympathetic nerve, and adrenal medulla, and it is currently believed that this enzyme is localized in the membrane of the amine storage granules. This enzyme usually disappears after chronic sympathetic denervation and therefore is believed present largely only in adrenergic neurons or adrenal chromaffin tissue. Dopamine β-hydroxylase does not show a high degree of substrate specificity and acts *in vitro* on a variety of substrates besides dopamine, oxidizing almost any phenylethylamine to its corresponding phenylethanolamine (i.e. tyramine $\longrightarrow$ octopamine, α-methyldopamine $\longrightarrow$ α-methylnorepinephrine). A number of the resultant, structurally analogous metabolites can replace norepinephrine at the noradrenergic nerve endings and function as "false neurotransmitters."

Dopamine-β-oxidase can be inhibited by a wide variety of compounds. The most effective are compounds which chelate copper: D-cysteine and L-cysteine, glutathione, mercaptoethanol, and coenzyme A. The inhibition can be reversed by addition of N-ethylmaleimide, which reacts with the sulfhydryl groups and interferes with the chelating properties of these substances. Copper chelating agents such as diethyldithiocarbamate have proved to be effective inhibitors both *in vivo* and *in vitro*. Thus it has been possible to treat animals with disulfuram and produce a reduction in brain norepinephrine and an elevation of brain dopamine. This manipulation might serve as a useful tool in the assessment of the relative roles of norepinephrine and dopamine in the central nervous system. However, in most cases, especially in the periphery, the dopamine which is not β-hydroxylated to norepinephrine does not accumulate to any great extent since it appears to be very rapidly deaminated by monoamine oxidase (MAO). The major increase, corresponding to the missing norepinephrine, is usually found in dopamine metabolites. Some recent work has indicated that endogenous inhibitors are found in tissue homogenates which when removed lead to a significant enhancement of dopamine-β-hydroxylase activity. It has been suggested that these inhibitors may have a role in the regulation of norepinephrine biosynthesis *in vivo* but it is also possible that they are artifacts of homogenization. There is little interest to develop more effective inhibitors of dopamine-β-hydroxylase since as much as 90 per cent inhibition of this enzyme *in vivo* by benzyloxyamine has no significant effect on the endogenous catecholamine levels.

Since dopamine-β-oxidase obtained from the bovine adrenal medulla can be prepared in a relatively pure form, it has been possible to produce a specific antibody to the enzyme. This antibody inactivates bovine dopamine-β-hydroxylase but does not appear to cross react with either DOPA decarboxylase or tyrosine hydroxylase. However, cross reactivity between dopamine-β-hydroxylase from human, guinea pig, and dog with the antibody against the bovine enzyme was observed and indicates that the enzymes from these various sources are probably structurally related. By coupling immunochemical techniques with fluorescence and electron microscopy, this antibody may help in localization of the enzyme in intact tissue.

Phenylethanolamine-N-methyl Transferase

In the adrenal medulla norepinephrine is N-methylated by the enzyme phenylethanolamine-N-methyltransferase to form epinephrine. This enzyme is largely restricted to the adrenal medulla although low levels of activity have been reported in heart and mammalian brain, especially in areas involved with olfaction. Like the decarboxylase, this enzyme also appears in the supernatant of homogenates. Demonstration of activity requires the presence of the methyl donor S-adenosyl methionine. The adrenal medullary enzyme shows poor substrate specificity and will transfer methyl groups to the nitrogen atom on a variety of β-hydroxylated amines. However, this adrenal enzyme is distinct from the nonspecific N-methyltransferase of rabbit lung, which in addition to N-methylating phenylethanolamine derivatives will also react with many normally occurring indoleamines and such diverse structures as phenylisopropylamine, aromatic amines, and phenanthrenes.

Synthesis Regulation

Knowledge concerning the various enzymes involved in the synthesis of dopamine, norepinephrine, and epinephrine have provided an excellent example of how extensive information of the individual components of a given biological system can contribute to a better understanding of its over-all function. Thus, once it was established that tyrosine hydroxylase was the rate-limiting step in the conversion of tyrosine to norepinephrine it did not take long to realize and to demonstrate experimentally that potent inhibitors of this initial step would effectively reduce tissue levels of norepinephrine. However, even as it becomes possible to understand more fully the chemistry and functional aspects of these enzymes under isolated conditions, this information still proves to be inadequate for a complete understanding of how, in fact, these enzymes function *in vivo*. It is necessary to have an appreciation of the cytological arrangement of the enzymes and cofactors within the neuron as well as some insight as to the external factors which may influence the activity of the neuron. Therefore it is becoming more and more important for neuropharmacologists to have a broad basic training and to take the time to try to interrelate the *in vivo* and *in vitro* data obtained experimentally to see if they can be correlated to provide a better understanding of the physiological control mechanisms involved.

It has been known for a long time that the degree of sympathetic activity does not influence the endogenous levels of norepinephrine; and it has been speculated that there must be some homeostatic mechanism whereby the level of transmitter is maintained at a relatively constant level in the sympathetic nerve endings despite the additional losses assumed to occur during enhanced sympathetic activity.

Recent experimental evidence now suggests that the ring hydroxylation of tyrosine to DOPA is regulated both *in vivo* and *in vitro* by sympathetic nerve activity: (1) Decentralization results in decreased conversion of tyrosine to catecholamines while the conversion of DOPA and dopamine to norepinephrine remains unaffected. (2) Increased sympathetic activity either *in vivo* or *in vitro* accelerates the formation of catecholamines from tyrosine but not from labeled DOPA. (3) Hypotensive drugs such as α-adrenergic blocking agents markedly increase the formation of norepinephrine from ^{14}C-tyrosine, an effect which can be blocked by ganglionic blocking agents. (4) Various phenothiazines, notably chlorpromazine, accelerate dopamine biosynthesis in the central nervous system presumably by causing a compensatory activation of dopaminergic neurons. In each of these cases the enzymatic biosynthetic step which is accelerated appears to be the rate-limiting hydroxylation of tyrosine. At least in the peripheral nervous system, this effect appears to be localized at the nerve terminals since stimulation of isolated sympathetic axons does not result in an acceleration of norepinephrine biosynthesis.

The actual mechanism(s) by which increased neuronal activity accelerates synthesis remains obscure. A number of interesting possibilities present themselves: (1) Since norepinephrine and dopamine can inhibit tyrosine hydroxylase *in vitro*, it has been suggested that depletion of a small pool of norepinephrine within the neuron strategically associated with the enzyme may stimulate tyrosine hydroxylase activity. Thus, the end product, norepinephrine or dopamine, could act as feedback inhibitors of the rate-limiting enzyme. (2) Increased nervous activity could directly increase the amount of enzyme (tyrosine hydroxylase) protein either by causing an increase in the synthesis of tyrosine hydroxylase or by inhibiting the normal turnover or destruction of the enzyme protein. (3) Neuronal activity could result in a release of a "local hormone" that influences enzymatic activity. (4) The ion fluxes during nerve stimulation could increase enzymatic activity possibly by an allosteric effect, resulting in a conformational change in the enzyme protein. (5) Nerve activation could alter the uptake of tyrosine into a specific site where it is selectively converted to DOPA.

Since short-term increases in neuronal activity, either *in vitro* or *in vivo* do not increase the amount of tyrosine hydroxylase, enzyme induction is unlikely to be responsible for the apparent increase in its activity. Although, after massive nerve stimulation of the vas deferens the post-stimulation increase in tyrosine to norepinephrine conversion can be antagonized by puromycin, this observation does not necessarily imply an increase in the synthesis of tyrosine hydroxylase. Thus, prolonged depolarization of this tissue with K^+ which results in more than a 100 per cent increase in norepinephrine biosynthesis *does not* result in an increase in tyrosine hydroxylase.

Allosteric activators of tyrosine hydroxylase have been considered, but experiments on partially purified adrenal medullary tyrosine hydroxylase showed no activation with various endogenous substances which might be expected to be released on nerve stimulation (that is, Na^+, K^+, Ca^{++}, acetylcholine, ATP, AMP, NAD^+, etc.). Furthermore, there is no evidence that the protein is, in fact, allosteric in nature. However, experiments conducted on an adrenal medullary enzyme may not apply to tyrosine hydroxylase isolated from sympathetic neurons. It is quite conceivable that tyrosine hydroxylase isolated from different sources could have substantially different properties.

Many experiments indirectly support the first possibility, that regulation occurs at the tyrosine hydroxylase step through a mechanism involving end product inhibition. Tyrosine hydroxylase from sympathetic nerves or adrenal medulla is inhibited *in vitro* by various catecholamines, apparently by competition with pteridine cofactor. *In vitro* addition of norepinephrine to the incubation media (10^{-6}M) blocks the nerve-stimulation-induced acceleration of norepinephrine biosynthesis in the vas deferens. Also, addition of norepinephrine to normal, nonstimulated vasa deferentia, brain slices, or heart slices results in a marked inhibition of norepinephrine biosynthesis. Additional studies have demonstrated that elevation of brain or heart catecholamine levels pharmacologically, by inhibition of monoamine oxidase, results in a substantial reduction of catecholamine biosynthesis in these tissues.

Recently, conditions other than direct nerve stimulation have been demonstrated to accelerate norepinephrine biosynthesis. Thus, the naturally occurring polypeptide angiotensin II, in amounts as low as 10^{-9}M, significantly increases norepinephrine formation. Also incubation of sympathetically innervated tissue in a high potassium medium results in a marked increase in catecholamine biosynthesis. This latter effect is apparent in tissue of both central and peripheral origin. Although the exact molecular mechanism in accelerating norepinephrine biosynthesis is still unknown at the present time, these agents may serve as effective tools for dissection of the molecular events involved in the regulation of norepinephrine biosynthesis.

It would be naïve to believe that catecholamine biosynthesis would not also be influenced by circulating hormones. In fact, steroid hormones will increase phenylethanolamine-*N*-methyltransferase activity both in the adrenal gland and in the central nervous system. Furthermore, thyroidectomy increases the conversion of ^{14}C-tyrosine to ^{14}C-norepinephrine. This finding suggests that normal degradation products of thyroid hormone (i.e. iodinated tyrosines) may be circulating in the bloodstream and acting as endogenous inhibitors of catecholamine biosynthesis. This, however, seems unlikely in normal individuals due to the presence of very active tissue dehalogenases. In certain patients with a defect in tissue dehalogenase this could become a reality, since it is known that in this instance iodotyrosines accumulate in the body and may reach levels expected to significantly inhibit tyrosine hydroxylase.

Even though tyrosine hydroxylase has been demonstrated to be rate limiting under most circumstances, this reaction may not remain rate limiting under all physiological conditions. Since there is a sequence of reactions, any one of these steps could assume a rate-limiting role depending upon the given pathological or pharmacologically induced situations. Thus, reserpine can transform the dopamine-β-hydroxylase step into the rate-limiting step presumably by blocking access of the substrate dopamine to the site of its conversion to norepinephrine. In fact, experiments utilizing the bovine splenic nerve granule as a model system have indicated that extragranular norepinephrine can effectively inhibit the uptake of dopamine into the granules and thus also inhibit the conversion of dopamine to norepinephrine. However, whether or not this sort of mechanism is functional *in vivo* (i.e. if high concentrations of cytoplasmic norepinephrine can inhibit the conversion of dopamine to norepinephrine) remains to be demonstrated.

Alternative Biosynthetic Pathways

The question has often been raised as to whether the sequence of enzymatic reactions described in detail above is in fact obligatory. Many attempts have been made to find alternative pathways *in vivo*, and to determine whether they are functionally important. Thus if labeled tyramine is administered to animals, both labeled norepinephrine and normetanephrine can be isolated in the urine. It has been very difficult to detect the conversion of tyramine to norepinephrine in sympathetically innervated tissue. However, the conversion of tyramine to dopamine has been demonstrated in liver microsomes. Therefore, it is possible that this conversion of tyramine to norepinephrine observed *in vivo* is a reflection of a metabolic reaction taking place in the liver rather than in the sympathetic neuron.

Turnover

The term "turnover" connotes the over-all rate at which the whole amine store within a given tissue is replaced. Thus, turnover rates are not necessarily identical with rates of biosynthesis. However, estimation of turnover rate can be used as an index to the functional state of various populations of sympathetic neurons, although not as an index of the synthetic capacity of the neurons.

Currently, many techniques are being utilized for the assessment of catecholamine turnover in both peripheral and central sympathetic neurons.

1. Turnover of norepinephrine has been estimated by measurement of the rate of decline of the specific activity of norepinephrine after a tracer dose of labeled amine is introduced into the endogenous pool. This technique has been applied both to peripheral and central neurons. In the case of the central nervous system the problem of penetration of the blood-brain barrier has been circumvented by administration of the labeled amine by intracisternal or intraventricular injections. This method for measurement of turnover, as one might expect, has a number of limitations. This method assumes that all the labeled norepinephrine found in the brain and in peripheral sympathetically innervated tissue is specifically retained by only the norepinephrine-containing neurons. This is not the case, since in addition to its retention in norepinephrine-containing neurons, labeled norepinephrine is also taken up and retained by a central network of dopamine-containing neurons in the central nervous system. In most cases this is not a serious limitation in the central nervous system

since, except for the dopamine neurons in the striatum, olfactory tubercle, and the median eminence, the remainder of the brain contains only a relatively small number of dopamine-containing neurons.

The isotope method assumes that only tracer amounts of labeled norepinephrine are introduced into the endogenous pool so that the size of the endogenous pool remains unaltered. This limitation has been largely overcome with the availability of norepinephrine of high specific activity and it is now possible to administer amounts of labeled norepinephrine which alter endogenous levels of amines by less than 5 per cent. Perhaps the greatest disadvantage of this method, which also applies to many other methods used to measure turnover, is the assumption that norepinephrine is stored in a single homogeneous pool with which the labeled norepinephrine mixes completely. In view of much biochemical, histochemical, and pharmacological evidence indicating more than one "pool" of catecholamines in sympathetic neurons, this assumption appears somewhat unlikely.

2. Another technique for measuring norepinephrine turnover involves following the disappearance rate of endogenous norepinephrine after inhibition of catecholamine biosynthesis by α-methyl-p-tyrosine or another potent inhibitor of tyrosine hydroxylase. This technique also suffers from several disadvantages. First, it involves measurement of an exponentially decreasing level of norepinephrine which is difficult to measure accurately in small tissue samples. Second, the required administration of large amounts of drugs (synthesis inhibitors) are almost certain to induce pharmacological actions aside from their "specific" action on tyrosine hydroxylase. Third, since turnover is being measured while endogenous levels of norepinephrine are being markedly depleted, this extensive depletion may in itself influence the normal control processes existing in the neuron.

3. An alternative isotopic method is to administer catecholamine precursors such as tyrosine or DOPA which are ultimately converted to labeled dopamine and norepinephrine. Catechol-

amine turnover is then determined by applying principles of steady state kinetics to the decline of norepinephrine and/or dopamine specific activities. The disadvantage of this method is that the results are complicated by the persistence of labeled catecholamine precursors in the circulation and tissues for considerable lengths of time after administration. This complication can be minimized to some extent by "chasing" the label with unlabeled precursor in order effectively to dilute the specific activity of the original agent.

4. Another isotope method involves the administration of labeled tyrosine and calculation of the rate of catecholamine synthesis from the rate of conversion of labeled tyrosine to labeled catecholamine. Provided that (a) endogenous catecholamine tissue levels remain unchanged, (b) that total tissue norepinephrine is derived from synthesis, and (c) that newly synthesized norepinephrine is not utilized (released or metabolized) preferentially, this technique provides a useful estimate of turnover.

5. More indirect methods for estimation of amine turnover in the central nervous system involve the measurement of amine metabolites released into ventricular perfusion fluids or their concentration changes in the cerebrospinal fluid (CSF). An advantage of this approach is its possible clinical application. It should be immediately pointed out that the degree of accumulation of a given metabolite in the central nervous system or cerebrospinal fluid is not necessarily an index of the quantity of metabolite formed, since most primary catecholamine metabolites can undergo further metabolism and be removed from the central nervous system or cerebrospinal fluid at different rates. Also drugs or various physiological conditions can alter routes of metabolism as well as rates of removal from the brain or cerebrospinal fluid independent of their effects on amine turnover. When estimation of metabolic end products of cerebral amine metabolism are used as indices to turnover, the interpretation remains extremely difficult, especially when alternative pathways may exist. Furthermore, many of the factors involved in the determination

TABLE 5.4. Effect of Various Procedures on Norepinephrine
Turnover in Rat Brain

Condition	Brain Region	$T \frac{1}{2}(hr)$	Turnover Rate $\mu g/gm/hr$
control	brain stem	5.4	0.094
pargyline		15.9	0.052
control	brain stem + mesencephalon	2.6	0.109
electroconvulsive shock treatment	brain stem + mesencephalon	2.3	0.152
control	brain stem + mesencephalon	2.6	0.148
paradoxical sleep rebound	brain stem + mesencephalon	1.5	0.270
control (24°C)	hypothalamus	5.09	
	brain less hypothalamus	2.72	
high temp. (32°C)	hypothalamus	1.77	
	brain less hypothalamus	2.18	
low temp. (9°C)	hypothalamus	5.78	
	brain less hypothalamus	2.91	

Data taken from Figs. 4 and 5, p. 53, L. L. Iversen and M. A. Simmonds, in: *Metabolism of Amines in the Brain.* (Ed. G. Hooper), Macmillan, 1969.

of steady state concentrations of these metabolites in either tissue or cerebrospinal fluid remain unknown.

The above methods for measurement of monoamine turnover have been applied in a number of experimental conditions. Some of the data obtained from various investigators is illustrated in Table 5-4. Pargyline, a monoamine oxidase inhibitor which causes an accumulation of monoamines within the brain, leads to a significant reduction in the turnover of norepinephrine. Electroconvulsive shock treatment and paradoxical sleep

TABLE 5-5. Turnover Time of Monoamine Stores of Various
Rat and Rabbit Tissue

Animal Species	Tissue	Turnover Time (in hours)	Synthesis Rate $\mu g/gm/hr$
Rat	heart NE	14.3	0.05
	brain NE	8.3	0.05
	brain DA	3.6	0.21
	brain 5-HT	1.2	0.50
Rabbit	caudate DA	3.0	2.85
	hypothalamic NE	5.3	0.46
	midbrain NE	5.0	0.12
	superior cervical ganglion NE	2.1	1.53
	iris NE	14.9	0.22
	salivary gland NE	10.0	0.12

Data taken from Table I and Table II in E. Costa and N. H. Neff, in
Proc. 3rd Int. Pharmacol. Meeting, 10, 15, 1968 Pergamon; and N. H.
Neff, and T. N. Tozer, Adv. Pharmacol., 6A, 97, 1968.

rebound lead to an increase in the turnover of brain stem +
mesencephalic norepinephrine. Exposure of rats to a high environmental temperature (32° C) which causes about a 3° rise
in rectal temperature produces a three-fold increase in the turnover of norepinephrine in the rat hypothalamus while it has
no significant effect on the rest of the brain. Lowering of the
environmental temperature, however, fails to cause a change
in the turnover of hypothalamic norepinephrine. Table 5-5
summarizes the turnover times of monoamine pools found in
various tissues of the rat and rabbit.

Storage

A great conceptual advance made in the study of catecholamines in the past fifteen years was the recognition that in almost

all tissues a large percentage of the norepinephrine present is located within highly specialized subcellular particles (colloquially referred to as "granules") in sympathetic nerve endings and chromaffin cells. Much of the norepinephrine in the central nervous system is also presumably located within similar particles. These granules contain adenosine triphosphate (ATP) in a molar ratio of catecholamine to ATP of about 4 : 1. Because of this perhaps fortuitous ratio, it is generally supposed that the anionic phosphate groups of ATP form a salt link with norepinephrine, which exists as a cation at physiological pH, and thereby serve as a means to bind the amines within the vesicles. Some such complex of the amines with ATP, with ATP associated with protein, or with protein directly is probable since the intravesicular concentration of amines, at least in the adrenal chromaffin granules and probably also in the splenic nerve granules (0.3 to 1.1 M), would be hypertonic if present in free solution and might be expected to lead to osmotic lysis of the vesicles.

The catecholamine storage vesicles in adrenal chromaffin and splenic nerve appear to have a number of general properties:

    a. they possess an outer limiting membrane;

    b. with appropriate fixation they possess an electron dense core when viewed in the electron microscope;

    c. they contain the enzyme dopamine-β-hydroxylase;

    d. they have a high concentration of catecholamine and ATP in a 4 : 1 ratio;

    e. chromaffin and splenic nerve granules contain a characteristic soluble protein (chromogranin) also suggested to be involved in the storage process;

    f. they contain Mg^{++} and Ca^{++} dependent ATPase.

The various types of vesicles found in neural tissue or chromaffin cells are summarized in Figure 5-14, which indicates their approximate size and distribution. A number of possible functions which have been proposed for the catecholamine storage vesicles are summarized below:

    a. They bind and store norepinephrine, thereby retarding its diffusion out of the neuron, and protect it from being

Neuronal and neuro-endocrine vesicles in mammals

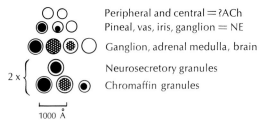

FIGURE 5-14. Size and electron microscopic appearance of the various types of synaptic vesicles, large granular vesicles, chromaffin granules, and neurosecretory granules found in various portions of the central and peripheral nervous system.

  destroyed by monoamine oxidase (MAO), which is considered to be intraneuronal;

b. they serve as a depot of transmitter which may be released upon the appropriate physiological stimulus;

c. they oxidize dopamine to norepinephrine;

d. they take up dopamine from the cytoplasm, protecting it from oxidation by monoamine oxidase.

It is generally believed that the vesicles are formed in the neuronal cell body and subsequently transported to the nerve terminal region. This assumption is based upon a number of findings:

a. protein biosynthesis has not been conclusively demonstrated in axons or nerve terminals;

b. following the depletion of norepinephrine by reserpine the amines first reappear within the perinuclear cytoplasm of the cell body;

c. when the axon of a sympathetic nerve is constricted, structures (mainly large granular vesicles containing norepinephrine) tend to accumulate at the proximal border.

Release

Much of the current knowledge regarding the release of catecholamines derives from the study of both adrenal medullary tissue and adrenergically innervated peripheral organs. Here it can be directly demonstrated that norepinephrine is released from the nerve terminals during periods of nerve stimulation and further that adrenergic fibers can sustain this output of transmitter during prolonged periods of stimulation, if synthesis and reuptake of the transmitter are not impaired. In the periphery it is possible to isolate the innervated end-organs, to collect a perfusate from the vascular system during nerve stimulation, and to analyze this for the presence and quantity of a given putative transmitter. However, we really know little of the mechanism by which axonal nerve impulses arriving at the terminal cause the release of norepinephrine (excitation-secretion coupling). Our best appreciation of the events comes from the possible analogous release of catecholamines from the adrenal medulla, which has been extensively studied. For a comprehensive review of this area the reader is referred to Douglas (1968). The mechanism of catecholamine release by the adrenal medulla is thought to take place as follows: with activity in the preganglionic fibers, acetylcholine is released and thought to combine with the plasma membrane of the chromaffin cells. This produces a change in membrane protein conformation altering the permeability of this membrane to Ca^{++} and other ions, which then move inward. The influx of Ca^{++} is believed to be the main stimulus responsible for the mobilization of the catecholamines and to cause their secretion. The current view is that the catecholamines are released from the chromaffin cell by a process of exocytosis, along with chromogranin, ATP, and a little dopamine-β-hydroxylase. Whether or not these cellular phenomena are applicable to the sympathetic nerve endings in general remains to be determined.

Teleologically, it appears rather unlikely that transmitter release from sympathetic nerve terminals does occur exclusively by a process of exocytosis. Exocytosis requires that the entire content of the granular vesicle be released (that is, catecholamine, ATP, and soluble protein). Since the nerve terminal region, as far as we know now, cannot sustain any sort of protein biosynthesis, high rates of axonal flow from the nerve cell body would be required to replenish the protein lost during the process of exocytosis. Alternatively, one might propose a "protein re-uptake" mechanism in order to recapture that protein released during the process of synaptic transmission. In peripheral nerve, release of norepinephrine has been shown to be frequency dependent within a physiological range of frequency. This release of norepinephrine, similar to the release of ACh, is Ca^{++}-dependent. Some evidence has also been presented which indicates that newly synthesized norepinephrine may be released preferentially. This preferential release is additional evidence to support the contention that norepinephrine exists in more than one pool within the sympathetic neuron.

It has been a great deal more difficult to demonstrate release of a putative transmitter from a given type of nerve ending in the central nervous system. Thus it is impossible to perfuse specific localized brain areas through their vascular system. In addition, it is also difficult but not necessarily impossible to stimulate a well-defined neuronal pathway within the brain. However, with the independent development of the push-pull cannula and the chemitrode, it has become possible to collect catecholamines from certain deep nuclear masses of the central nervous system. In addition, cortical cups, ventricular perfusions, brain slices, and isolated spinal cords have been used to demonstrate release of putative transmitters, including norepinephrine and dopamine from central nervous system tissue. All of these physiological techniques for studying release have some disadvantages and limitations and are somewhat gross and indirect (see Chapters 2 and 3). Nevertheless they do represent increasing sophistication in research on release occurring in the central nervous system.

Metabolism

The metabolism of exogenously administered or endogenous catecholamines differs markedly from that of acetylcholine in that the speed of degradation of the amines is considerably slower than that of the ACh-ACh-esterase system. The major mammalian enzymes of importance in the metabolic degradation of catecholamines are monoamine oxidase and catechol-*O*-methyltransferase (COMT) (Fig. 5-15). Monoamine oxidase is an enzyme which converts catecholamines to their corresponding aldehydes. This aldehyde intermediate is rapidly metabolized, usually by oxidation by the enzyme aldehyde dehydrogenase to the corresponding acid. In some circumstances, the aldehyde is reduced to the alcohol or glycol by aldehyde reductase. Neither of these latter enzymes has been extensively studied in neuronal tissue. Monoamine oxidase is a particle-bound protein, localized largely in the outer membrane of mitochondria, although a partial microsomal localization cannot be excluded. There is also some evidence for a riboflavin-like material in monoamine oxidase from liver mitochondria. Monoamine oxidase is usually considered to be an intraneuronal enzyme, but it occurs in abundance extraneuronally. In fact, most experiments indicate that chronic denervation of a sympathetic end-organ leads only to a relatively small reduction in monoamine oxidase, suggesting that the greater proportion of this enzyme is, in fact, extraneuronal. However, it is the intraneuronal enzyme which seems to be important in catecholamine metabolism. Dopamine appears to be a better substrate for monoamine oxidase than either epinephrine or norepinephrine, and large amounts of the deaminated metabolites of dopamine (dihydroxyphenylacetic acid and homovanillic acid) are excreted daily in human urine. It has been speculated that under certain circumstances this enzyme could serve to regulate norepinephrine biosynthesis by controlling the amount of substrate, dopamine, available to the enzyme dopamine-β-hydroxylase. Monoamine oxidase is not an exclusive catabolic enzyme for the catecholamines since it also oxidatively deaminates other biogenic amines such as 5-hydroxytryptamine, tryptamine, and tyramine. The intraneuronal localization of monoamine oxidase in mitochondria or other structures suggests that this would limit its action to amines that are present in a free (unbound) form in the axoplasm. Here, monoamine oxidase can act on amines that have been taken up by the axon before they are granule-bound, or it

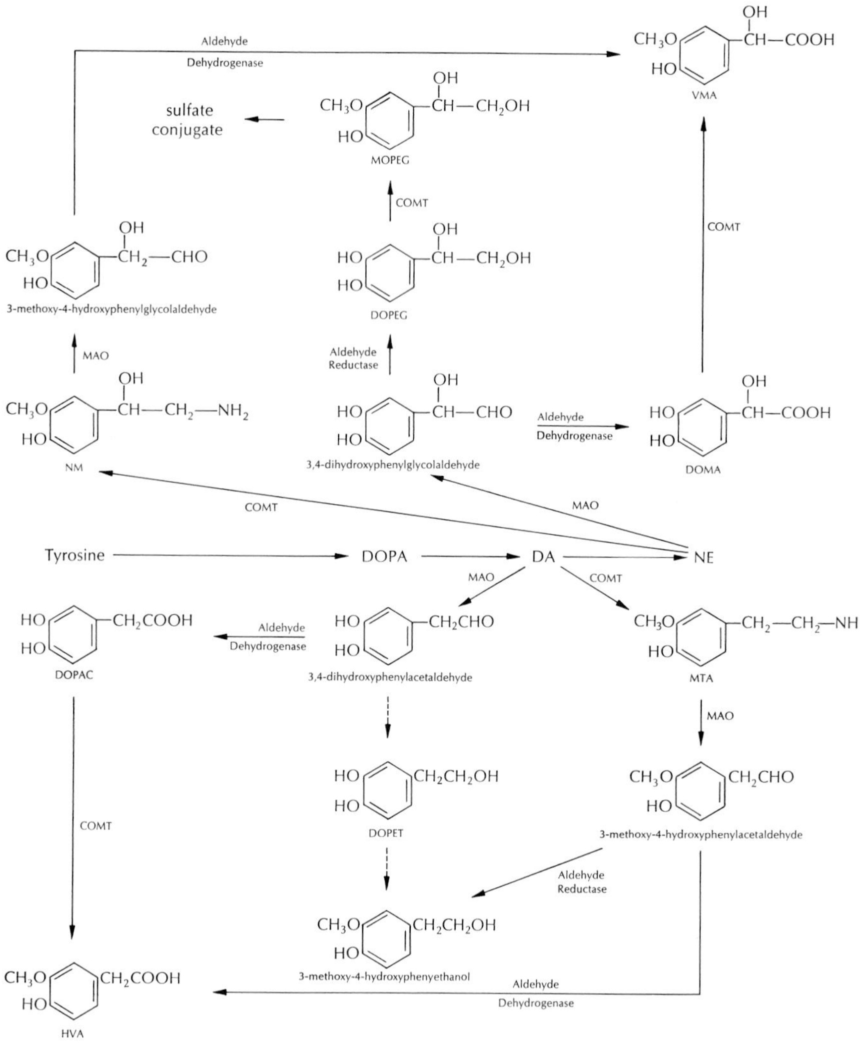

Aldehyde Dehydrogenase

sulfate conjugate

CH_3O, HO — CH—CH_2OH — MOPEG

CH_3O, HO — CH—$COOH$ — VMA

COMT

COMT

CH_3O, HO — CH_2—CHO — 3-methoxy-4-hydroxyphenylglycolaldehyde

HO, HO — CH—CH_2OH — DOPEG

COMT

MAO

Aldehyde Reductase

CH_3O, HO — CH—CH_2—NH_2 — NM

HO, HO — CH—CHO — 3,4-dihydroxyphenylglycolaldehyde

Aldehyde Dehydrogenase

HO, HO — CH—$COOH$ — DOMA

COMT

MAO

Tyrosine ———→ DOPA ——→ DA ——→ NE

HO, HO —CH_2COOH — DOPAC

Aldehyde Dehydrogenase

HO, HO —CH_2CHO — 3,4-dihydroxyphenylacetaldehyde

MAO

COMT

CH_3O, HO —CH_2—CH_2—NH — MTA

MAO

HO, HO —CH_2CH_2OH — DOPET

CH_3O, HO —CH_2CHO — 3-methoxy-4-hydroxyphenylacetaldehyde

Aldehyde Reductase

COMT

CH_3O, HO —CH_2CH_2OH — 3-methoxy-4-hydroxyphenylethanol

Aldehyde Dehydrogenase

CH_3O, HO —CH_2COOH — HVA

can even act on amines that are released from the granules before they pass out through the axonal membrane. Interestingly, the latter possibility seems physiologically minor, since monoamine oxidase inhibition does not potentiate the effects of nerve stimulation.

Figure 5-15. Dopamine and Norepinephrine Metabolism. The following abbreviations are used: DOPA, dihydroxyphenylalanine; DA, dopamine; NE, norepinephrine; DOMA, 3,4-dihydroxymandelic acid; DOPAC, 3,4-dihydroxyphenylacetic acid; DOPEG, 3,4-dihydroxyphenylglycol; DOPET, 3,4-dihydroxyphenylethanol; MOPET, 3-methoxy-4-hydroxy-phenylethanol; MOPEG, 3-methoxy-4-hydroxy-phenylglycol; HVA, homovanillic acid; VMA, 3-methoxy-4-hydroxy-mandelic acid; NM, normetanephrine; MTA, 3-methoxytyramine; MAO, monoamine oxidase; COMT, catechol-O-methyltransferase; Dashed arrows indicated steps which have not been firmly established.

The second enzyme of importance in the catabolism of catecholamines is catechol-O-methyltransferase discovered by Axelrod in 1957. This enzyme is a relatively nonspecific enzyme which catalyzes the transfer of methyl groups from S-adenosylmethionine to the *m*-hydroxyl group of catecholamines and various other catechol compounds. Catechol-O-methyltransferase is found in the cytoplasm of most animal tissue, being particularly abundant in kidney and liver. A substantial amount of this enzyme is also found in the central nervous system and in various sympathetically innervated organs. The precise cellular localization of catechol-O-methyltransferase has not been determined although it has been suggested (with little foundation) to function extraneuronally. The purified enzyme requires S-adenosylmethionine and Mg^{++} ions for activity. As with monoamine oxidase, inhibition of catechol-O-methyltransferase activity does not markedly potentiate the effects of sympathetic nerve stimulation, although in some tissue it tends to prolong the response. Therefore, neither monoamine oxidase nor catechol-O-methyltransferase would seem to be the primary mechanism for terminating the action of norepinephrine liberated at sympathetic nerve terminals.

Uptake

When sympathetic postganglionic nerves are stimulated at frequencies low enough to be comparable to those encountered physiologically, very little intact norepinephrine overflows into the circulation, suggesting that local inactivation is very efficient. This local inactivation is not significantly blocked when catechol-O-methyltransferase or monoamine oxidase or both are inhibited, and it is believed to involve mainly uptake or (re-uptake) by sympathetic neurons.

Considerable attention has been directed to the role of tissue uptake mechanisms in the physiological inactivation of catecholamines. But only in recent years has this concept received direct experimental support, although a number of earlier findings had in fact suggested that catecholamines might be inactivated by some sort of nonmetabolic processes. For example, almost forty years ago Burn suggested the possibility that exogenous norepinephrine might be taken up in storage sites in peripheral tissue. About twenty years ago it was demonstrated that an increase in the catecholamine content of cat and dog heart occurred after administration of norepinephrine and epinephrine *in vivo*. However, in view of the very high doses (mg) employed in these experiments, the significance of the findings remained questionable. It was really not until labeled catecholamines with high specific activity became available that similar experiments using doses of norepinephrine comparable to those likely to be encountered under physiological circumstances could be performed. Uptake studies of this nature carried out *in vivo* have indicated that approximately 40 to 60 per cent of a relatively small intravenous dose of norepinephrine is metabolized enzymatically by catechol-O-methyltransferase and monoamine oxidase, while the remainder is inactivated by uptake into various tissues. This uptake appears to be extremely rapid, and in most cases the magnitude of the uptake is related to the density of sympathetic innervation and the proportion of cardiac output received by the tissue in question. Thus, after administration of ^{3}H-norepinephrine *in vivo*, the greatest uptake and binding occur in tissues such as spleen and heart. The brain is also capable of taking up norepinephrine but, since the uptake from the circulation is prevented by the blood-brain barrier, efficient uptake can only be observed in brain slices, minces, or brain synapto-somes exposed to norepinephrine or when the labeled amines are administered intraventricularly or intracisternally.

A large amount of data from the past few years suggests that the major site of this uptake (and subsequent binding) ac-tually occurs in sympathetic nerves. This evidence can be sum-marized as follows:

   a. In most cases norepinephrine uptake correlates directly with the density of sympathetic innervation (or the en-dogenous content of norepinephrine) providing that suffi-cient allowance is made for differences in regional blood flow to various tissues.
   b. In tissues without a normal sympathetic nerve supply the ability to take up exogenous catecholamines is severely impaired. This can be demonstrated by surgical sympa-thectomy, chemical sympathectomy, or immunosympa-thectomy.
   c. Labeled norepinephrine taken up by heart, spleen, artery, vein, or other tissues can be subsequently released by sympathetic nerve stimulation.
   d. Autoradiographic studies at the electron microscope level have directly localized labeled catecholamines within the neuronal elements of the tissue.
   e. Fluorescence microscopy has also provided equally direct evidence for the localization of norepinephrine uptake to sympathetic nerves.

A number of studies demonstrate that the uptake of cate-cholamines is active as it proceeds against a concentration gra-dient. For example, slices or minces of heart, spleen, and brain can concentrate norepinephrine to levels five to eight times those in the incubation medium. In intact tissues even greater concen-tration ratios between tissue and medium may be obtained. In isolated rat heart perfused with Krebs solution containing 10 ng/ml of norepinephrine, Iversen finds concentrations of labeled norepinephrine rise thirty to forty times above that present in the perfusion medium. If we assume that norepinephrine uptake occurs almost exclusively into cardiac sympathetic neurons, the uptake process clearly has an exceptionally high affinity for norepinephrine. In fact, the actual concentration ratios between exogenous norepinephrine accumulated within the sympathetic neurons and that present in the medium could approach 10,000 : 1. This uptake process is a saturable membrane transport process dependent upon temperature and requiring energy. The stereochemically preferred substrate is L-norepinephrine; furthermore, norepinephrine is taken up more efficiently than its N-substituted derivatives. This process is sodium dependent and can be blocked by inhibition of Na, K-activated ATPase. In fact, most evidence suggests that catecholamine uptake is mediated by some sort of active membrane transport mechanism located in the axonal membrane of postganglionic sympathetic neurons.

AXONAL TRANSPORT

The early estimates of the rate of axoplasmic transport by Weiss, based both on the rate of regeneration of axons and on nerve constriction experiments suggested that the total mass of axonal material is transported distally at a rate of approximately 1 mm/day. More recent studies employing the use of radioactive substances and autoradiography have evaluated the transport of individual components of the axoplasm. Numerous demonstrations indicate some proteins are transported at rates of approximately 1 mm/day; but, in addition, a heterogeneity of transport rates of some axoplasmic constituents, ranging up to 10 cm/day and even up to 1 meter/day, have also been reported. Many of these experiments have been concerned with the axonal transport of catecholamines, as described by Dahlström and her colleagues in Sweden. They found that ligated sympathetic nerves accumulate norepinephrine above the ligation indicating a proximo-distal transport of amine-containing particles from the nerve cell body. Not only was this accumulation studied biochemically but also histochemical fluorescence observations of the zone of constriction were made at different times after ligation.

It was found that when a sympathetic axon is crushed or ligated, there is an almost immediate accumulation of norepinephrine on the cell body side of the ligature or crush. After 12 to 24 hours there is a marked accumulation of norepinephrine in the segment proximal to the crush, with only a weak or small accumulation in the distal segment. The increase in norepinephrine on the proximal side proceeds linearly up to about 48 hours, at which time it tends to level off. Pharmacological treatment with reserpine indicated that the accumulated norepinephrine is stored within the granules. From the content of norepinephrine in 1 cm segments of nonligated axon and the rate of accumulation of norepinephrine in the 1 cm segment proximal to the ligature, the velocity of the transport of the norepinephrine-containing particles was calculated to be about 5 mm/hr in the rat, 10 mm/hr in the cat, and 2-3 mm/hr in the rabbit.

Dahlström also made tandem constrictions by using two ligatures and found that the accumulation of norepinephrine was considerably larger above the proximal ligation than above the distal ligation. In the part of the nerve between the two ligatures, the total norepinephrine did not exceed the amount in a normal unligated nerve segment of the identical length, suggesting that local synthesis was probably not responsible to any extent for the accumulation normally observed. Other experiments conducted in the central nervous system have suggested that the transport rate in this tissue is about 0.5 mm/hr.

Even in view of these fairly rapid rates of transport of catecholamine storage granules it seems unlikely that this transport process serves to replace transmitter normally lost during nerve activity. More probably this transport serves to replace the granular protein structure which houses or binds the catecholamine, and turns over at a slower rate than that of the amines.

NEUROTRANSMITTER ROLE

On the basis of many experiments demonstrating that norepinephrine is synthesized and stored in sympathetic neurons, that it is released in significant quantities in response to sympathetic nerve stimulation, that it produces effector organ responses identical to those produced by sympathetic nerve stimulation, and that drugs which antagonize the action of exogenous norepinephrine also block the effect of sympathetic nerve stimulation of the organ in question, it has been accepted by most investigators that norepinephrine is in fact the sympathetic neurotransmitter in the mammalian peripheral sympathetic nervous system.

Although it is quite well accepted that norepinephrine acts as a neurotransmitter in peripheral noradrenergic nerve terminals, the evidence that norepinephrine acts as a central neurotransmitter is not nearly so compelling. As described in Chapter 2 the central nervous system obviously presents an immediate obstacle to cellular investigations, namely, one of inaccessibility. Not only is the central nervous system of mammals relatively inaccessible but it does not have the clear-cut focal synaptic regions found in the peripheral nervous system. The cell bodies, dendrites, and axons of central neurons are usually studded with synaptic boutons. This, of course, provides the investigator with a totally heterogeneous system of chemical and perhaps electrical inputs in close proximity to each other, making it difficult to evaluate events taking place at a particular type of nerve ending. A number of criteria, of course, must be fulfilled before it is possible to accept a putative transmitter candidate as a true neurotransmitter at a given synaptic junction. These criteria have been reviewed in Chapter 2. Many of the proposed criteria for neurotransmitters have been satisfactorily fulfilled by norepinephrine and dopamine in the mammalian central nervous system. The major difficulties in transmitter identification in the central nervous system have been in demonstrating the release of the transmitter and in comparing the postsynaptic effects of presynaptic nerve stimulation and those obtained upon application of the putative transmitter to the postsynaptic receptor. If one imposes the most stringent criteria for evaluating release, it is necessary to demonstrate that the putative transmitter is released into the diffusable volume of the synaptic cleft in response to stimulation and depolarization of a given nerve terminal. At present no micromethod has yet been devised by which it is possible to study release at this fine level of refinement in the central nervous system. If one is not so critical, release of monoamines can be demonstrated by a number of experimental techniques from central nervous system tissue. For example norepinephrine is released from brain slices by gross nonspecific electrical stimulation. It has also been shown that stimulation of an isolated spinal cord produces a release of some norepinephrine and 5-hydroxytryptamine into the media.

With even less stringent criteria of acceptibility, perfusion of the lateral ventricles of cats reveals detectable amounts of dopamine, norepinephrine, and their metabolites in the cerebrospinal fluid after periods of low level stimulation of certain brain areas. Here, however, we must assume that the putative transmitter released from certain nerve endings within the brain escapes the recapture process and diffuses through the brain substance proper to be detected eventually in the cerebrospinal fluid. More "refined" techniques such as push-pull cannulae and chemitrodes have also provided evidence for norepinephrine and dopamine release in both acute and chronically implanted animals. This latter release is also enhanced by electrical stimulation or by certain drugs. A number of even less direct techniques has often been used to demonstrate release *in vivo*. Thus, fluorescence histochemical experiments demonstrating depletion of nerve terminal fluorescence have been used as an index of release. Similarly, biochemical studies demonstrating depletion of catecholamines have been used as an index of release. However, other plausible explanations of this depletion such as acceleration of catabolism should also be considered.

It has also been difficult in the central nervous system to demonstrate that administration of an exogenous quantity of a putative transmitter produces the same effect as nerve terminal depolarization and that drugs which block the action of this natural transmitter at the receptor also exhibit the same degree of sensitivity toward the putative transmitter. Microiontophoresis has provided a powerful tool toward this end.

By means of this technique these criteria have been satisfied for the olfactory bulb and for the caudate nucleus. In the olfactory bulb norepinephrine may be a mediator of a recurrent inhibitory synaptic pathway since: (a) iontophoretically applied norepinephrine depresses spontaneous activity; (b) this effect as well as depression due to synaptic inhibition can be blocked by dibenamine, an α-adrenergic blocking agent; (c) synaptic inhibition is reduced when catecholamines are depleted by pretreating animals with reserpine and α-methyl tyrosine; (d) norepinephrine-containing nerve endings appear to be restricted to the layer in the olfactory bulb where synaptic inhibition is most easily demonstrated.

In the caudate nucleus and spinal cord, areas rich in catecholamine-containing nerve endings, α-receptor blocking drugs are also capable of blocking the response to iontophoretically applied catecholamines. Further, in the caudate nucleus this response to the catecholamines is identical with that resulting from stimulation of the substantia nigra where dopamine-containing nerve endings are thought to arise.

In almost all cases the response of single neurons to norepinephrine and dopamine is a depression of spontaneous activity. In the cerebellum the norepinephrine response appears to be mediated by cyclic AMP.

It is clear that so far a critical assessment of neurotransmitter function for norepinephrine and dopamine in the central nervous system is almost completely lacking due largely to technical deficiencies. However, a great deal of evidence does suggest the possibility that both norepinephrine and dopamine do play such a role in the central nervous system.

PHARMACOLOGY OF CATECHOLAMINE NEURONS

In this section we will focus on the pharmacology of the central nervous system discussing possible sites of drug involvement in the life cycle of the catecholamines. Figure 5-16 depicts a schematic model of a noradrenergic nerve varicosity.

Site-1—Precursor transport. As noted earlier there appears to be an active uptake or transport of tyrosine as well as other aromatic

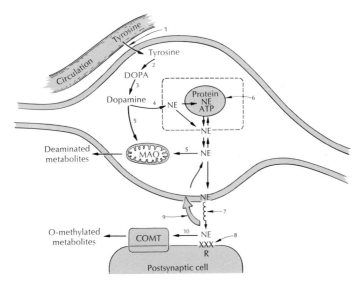

FIGURE 5-16. Schematic model of noradrenergic neuron.

amino acids into the central nervous system. In addition it is also probable that tyrosine is actively taken up by adrenergic neurons both in the periphery and in the central nervous system. At present we have no pharmacologic agent which specifically antagonizes the uptake of tyrosine into the brain or into the catecholamine-containing neuron. However, it is known that various aromatic amino acids will compete with each other for transport into the central nervous system. This competition might become important under a pathological situation in which blood aromatic amino acids are elevated. Thus in phenylketonuria, when plasma levels of phenylalanine are elevated to about 10^{-3}M, it might be expected that tyrosine and tryptophan uptake into the brain might be diminished.

Site-2—Tyrosine hydroxylase. The conversion of tyrosine to DOPA is the rate limiting step in this biosynthetic pathway and thus is the step most susceptible to pharmacological manipulation. The various classes of tyrosine hydroxylase inhibitors were considered earlier in this chapter. α-methyl-*p*-tyrosine, an effective inhibitor of tyrosine hydroxylase both *in vivo* and *in vitro*, is one of the few tyrosine hydroxylase inhibitors which has been employed clinically and found to be effective in the treatment of pheochromocytomas; it is of little or no value in the treatment of essential hypertension.

Sites-3 and 4—DOPA-decarboxylase and dopamine-β-oxidase. Potent inhibitors of DOPA-decarboxylase and dopamine-β-oxidase do exist but they are generally not effective *in vivo* in reducing tissue concentrations of catecholamines.

Due to the nonspecificity of these two enzymes (see above) as well as the relatively nonspecific vesicular storage sites, certain drugs or even amines or amine precursors in foodstuff can be synthesized to phenylethylamine derivatives with a catechol or a β-hydroxyl group and taken up and stored in the storage vesicles. These compounds can subsequently be released by sympathetic nerves, in part replacing some of the norepinephrine normally released by sympathetic impulses. Since these "false neurotransmitters" are less potent in their action, replacement of some of the endogenous, releasable pool of norepinephrine with these agents results in a diminished sympathetic response. Thus a drug such as α-methyldihydroxyphenylalanine, which is converted in the sympathetic neuron to α-methyl-norepinephrine, replaces a portion of the endogenous norepinephrine and itself can be subsequently released as a "false transmitter." The false transmitter theory also has been used to explain the hypotensive action of various monoamine oxidase inhibitors. Tyramine, an endogenous metabolite which is normally disposed of by monoamine oxidase in the liver and other tissues, is no longer rapidly deaminated in the presence of monoamine oxidase inhibitors and thus can be converted to the β-hydroxylated derivative octopamine which then accumulates in sympathetic neurons. Upon activation of these nerves, octopamine is released and acts as a false neurotransmitter, producing a resultant decrease in sympathetic tone (observed with monoamine oxidase inhibitors). "False neurotransmitter" can also be formed in the brain. However at the present time the action of these agents is unclear.

Site-5—Metabolic degradation by monoamine oxidase. The mono-amine oxidase inhibitors comprise quite a heterogeneous group of drugs which have in common the ability to block the oxidative deamination of various biogenic amines. These agents all produce marked increases in tissue amine concentrations. These compounds are in most cases employed clinically for the treatment of depression. However, some of these agents are used for the treatment of hypertension and angina pectoris. In the case of monoamine oxidase inhibitors, it should be immediately pointed out that while these drugs inhibit monoamine oxidase, there is no firmly established correlation between monoamine oxidase inhibition and therapeutic effect. In fact, it is generally well appreciated that monoamine oxidase inhibitors inhibit not only enzymes involved in oxidative deamination of monoamines but in addition many other enzymes unrelated to monoamine oxidase such as succinic dehydrogenase, dopamine β-oxidase, 5-hydroxytryptophan decarboxylase, choline dehydrogenase, and diamine oxidase.

Site-6—Storage. A number of drugs, most notably the Rauwolfia alkaloids, interfere with the storage of monoamines by blocking the uptake of amine into the storage granules or by disrupting the binding of the amines. Thus drugs interfering with the storage mechanism will cause amines to be released intraneuronally. Amines released intraneuronally appear to be preferentially metabolized by monoamine oxidase.

Site-7—Release. The release of catecholamines is dependent upon Ca^{++} ions. Thus, in an *in vitro* system it is possible to block release by lowering the Ca^{++} concentration of the medium. Although drugs such as bretylium act to inhibit the release of norepinephrine in the peripheral nervous system, this drug does not easily penetrate the brain and thus has little or no effect on central monoaminergic neurons. γ-hydroxybutyrate, a naturally occurring metabolite of brain (see Chapter 7), when administered in anesthetic doses to rats produces a large increase in brain dopamine, largely by effectively blocking the release or utilization of dopamine. The action of the agent as a drug appears to be quite specific in that it has little effect on other brain monoamines such as norepinephrine or 5-hydroxytryptamine.

Site-8—Interaction with receptors. α and β adrenergic blocking agents are effective in the peripheral nervous system. These agents block both the effects of sympathetic nerve stimulation and the action of exogenously administered norepinephrine. Some of these agents also have central activity. However, the ability of the adrenergic blocking agents specifically to inhibit adrenergic transmission or the action of exogenous sympathomimetic amines on the central nervous system has not always been convincingly demonstrated.

Site-9—Re-uptake. Drugs such as cocaine, imipramine, amitrypty-line, and other related trycyclic antidepressants are effective inhibitors of norepinephrine uptake both at peripheral and central sites. Pharmacological intervention at these sites makes more norepinephrine available to the receptor and thus tends to potentiate adrenergic transmission. The dopamine-containing neurons in the brain appear to possess a somewhat different uptake mechanism in that they show a preferential affinity for dopamine. In addition, this uptake is not strongly inhibited by the tricyclic antidepressants.

Site-10—Catechol-O-methyltransferase. Catechol-O-methyltransferase can be inhibited by pyrogallol or various tropolone derivatives. Inhibition of this enzyme in most sympathetically innervated tissue such as heart does not significantly potentiate the effects of nerve stimulation. In vascular tissue, however, inhibition of this enzyme does lead to a significant prolongation of the response to nerve stimulation.

Catecholamine Theory of Affective Disorders

The catecholamines play a fairly well-established role in the periphery with regard to stress and emotional behavior. By contrast their suggested role in the central nervous system in affective disorders is still quite speculative although evidence for the involvement of these agents is becoming increasingly compelling.

A catecholamine hypothesis of affective disorder has arisen which states that, in general, behavioral depression may be related to a deficiency of catecholamine (usually norepinephrine) at functionally important central adrenergic receptors, while mania results from excess catecholamine. While substantial experimental work bears on this proposal it must be kept in mind that most of the experiments on which this hypothesis is based derive from "normal" animals. Secondly, from a nosological standpoint, depression itself is rather ill defined. In fact, Giarman has suggested that "nosologically it might be fair to compare the depressive syndrome with the anemias. Certainly, no self-respecting hematologist would subscribe to a unitary biochemical explanation for all of the anemias."

The original impetus for formulation of the catecholamine hypothesis was the finding that various monoamine oxidase inhibitors, notably iproniazid, acted clinically as mood elevators or antidepressants. Shortly thereafter it was found that this class of compounds also produced marked increases in brain amine levels. By the same token, reserpine, a potent tranquilizer which causes depletion of brain amines, sometimes produces a serious depressed state (clinically indistinguishable from endogenous depression) and even suicidal attempts in man. Although both classes of drugs altered brain levels of catecholamines and serotonin quite equally, the fact that precursors of catecholamine biosynthesis, notably DOPA, could reverse most of the reserpine-induced symptomology in animals has tended to bias many in favor of the catecholamine theory (see Chapter 6). In general, many pharmacological studies appear to implicate the catecholamines as the amines involved in affective disorders. However, it must be realized that a great deal more work has been done on norepinephrine than on other transmitter candidates. In fact, by no means does the available evidence obtained for the involvement of norepinephrine rule out the participation of dopamine, 5-hydroxytryptamine, or other putative transmitters in similar events.

The three general classes of drugs most commonly used to treat various depressive disorders are the monoamine oxidase inhibitors, the tricyclic antidepressants, and the psychomotor stimulants of which amphetamine was the prototype. All of these pharmacological agents appear to interact with catecholamines in a way which is consistent with the catecholamine hypothesis.

The amphetamines, even if one considers all the suggested modes of action—(a) partial agonist, mimicking action of norepinephrine at receptor, (b) inhibition of re-uptake, (c) inhibition of monoamine oxidase, (d) displacement of norepinephrine, releasing it onto receptors—appear to exert an action compatible with the hypothesis above since the net result of all of these actions would be a temporary increase of norepinephrine at the receptor or a direct stimulatory action at the receptor. Upon administration of chronic or high doses of amphetamine it is possible to produce an eventual depletion of brain norepinephrine perhaps due to a displacement of norepinephrine in the neuron and/or an inhibition of synthesis. This chronic depletion may relate to the clinical observation of amphetamine tolerance or to the well-known poststimulation depression or fatigue observed after chronic administration of this class of drugs.

The tricyclic antidepressants may exert their action by inhibiting the catecholamine axonal membrane pump (see above). In support of this proposal the tricyclic antidepressants potentiate the peripheral autonomic effects of exogenous norepinephrine, the adrenergic responses elicited by both pre- and postganglionic sympathetic nerves stimulation and the central effects of DOPA and amphetamine. In addition, their action is prevented by selective depletion of brain amines with α-methyl-para-tyrosine as well as by administration of adrenergic blocking agents. While these findings are of course also consistent with the catecholamine hypothesis, the tricyclics do not affect this system exclusively. Thus, some of the tricyclic agents, notably imipramine, also potentiate peripheral and central effects of serotonin; they also have both central and peripheral anticholinergic actions.

The action of the monoamine oxidase inhibitors also supports the catecholamine hypothesis. All these agents inhibit an enzyme responsible for the metabolism of norepinephrine and various other amines (5-hydroxytryptamine, dopamine, tyramine, tryptamine). This inhibition results in a marked increase in the intraneuronal levels of norepinephrine. Presumably, according to the conceptual model of the adrenergic neuron presented above, this interneuronal norepinephrine might eventually diffuse out of the neuron and reach receptor cells, thus overcoming the presumed deficiency. A similar mechanism may also explain the antagonism of reserpine-induced sedation with monoamine oxidase inhibitors, since there will be a replenishment of the norepinephrine deficiency initially caused by reserpine.

Lithium, one of the main agents used in the treatment of mania has also been studied with regard to its action on the life cycle of the catecholamines. Interestingly, pretreatment with lithium blocks the stimulus-induced release of norepinephrine from rat brain slices. Other investigators have suggested that lithium may facilitate re-uptake of norepinephrine. If the inhibition of release observed in stimulated brain slices is due to a facilitated recapture mechanism, then the mechanism of action of lithium would be the exact opposite of that of the antidepressant drugs, as would be expected according to the catecholamine hypothesis.

SELECTED REFERENCES

Acheson, G. H. (1965). Second catecholamine symposium, *Pharmacol. Rev.* *18*, 1.

Aghajanian, G. K., and R. H. Roth (1970). γ-Hydroxybutyrate-induced increase in brain dopamine: Localization by fluorescence microscopy (*J. Pharmacol.* in press).

Akert, K., and P. G. Waser (1969). Mechanisms of synaptic transmission. *Progress in Brain Res.* *31*, 1.

Björkland, A., B. Ehinger, and B. Falck (1968). A method for differentiating dopamine from norepinephrine in tissue sections by microspectrofluorometry. *J. Histochem. Cytochem.* *16*, 263.

Bloom, F. E. (1970). The fine structural localization of biogenic monoamines in nervous tissue. *International Rev. Neurobiology*, in press.

Bloom, F. E., and N. J. Giarman (1968). Current status of neurotransmitters. *Ann. Rep. Medicinal Chem.*, Chap. 25, Academic Press, New York.

Bloom, F. E., and N. J. Giarman (1968). Physiologic and pharmacologic considerations of biogenic amines in the nervous system. *Ann. Rev. Pharmacol.* *8*, 229.

Dahlström, A. and J. Häggendal (1966). Studies on the transport and life-span of amine storage granules in a peripheral adrenergic neuron system. *Acta physiol. Scand.* 67, 278.

Douglas, W. W. (1968). Stimulus-secretion coupling: The concept and clues from chromaffin and other cells. *Brit. J. Pharmacol.* *34*, 451.

Euler, U. S. von (1956). *Noradrenaline*. Charles C. Thomas, Springfield, Ill.

Falck, B., and A. Torp (1961). A fluorescence method for histochemical demonstration of norepinephrine in adrenal medulla. *Med. Exp.* *5*, 429.

Giarman, N. J. (1968). Modes and sites of action of psychic energizers. *Mind as a Tissue*. Hoeber, New York, p. 123.

140

Hooper, G. (1969). *Metabolism of Amines in the Brain.* Macmillan, London.

Hornykiewicz, O. (1966). Dopamine and brain function. *Pharmacol. Rev. 18,* 925.

Iversen, L. L. (1967). *The Uptake and Storage of Noradrenaline in Sympathetic Nerves.* Harvard University Press, Cambridge, Mass.

Kopin, I. J. (1968). False adrenergic transmitters. *Ann. Rev. Pharmacol. 8,* 377.

Schildkraut, J. J. (1969). Neuropsychopharmacology and the affective disorders. *New England J. Med. 281.*

Stjärne, L. (1964). Studies of catecholamine uptake, storage and release mechanisms. *Acta physiol. scand. 62,* Suppl. 228.

Udenfriend, S. (1962). *Fluorescence Assay in Biology and Medicine.* Academic Press, New York.

Vane, J. R. (1969). The release and fate of vaso-active hormones in the circulation. *Brit. J. Pharmacol. 35,* 209.

Van Orden, L. S., J-M. Schaefer, J. P. Burk, and F. V. Lodoen (1970). Differentiation of norepinephrine storage compartments in peripheral adrenergic neurons. *J. Pharmacol.* (in press).

6 | Serotonin (5-hydroxytryptamine)

Historical Introduction

Of all the neurotransmitter substances we shall discuss, serotonin is the one whose history is most intimately involved with neuropsychopharmacology. Since the middle of the nineteenth century, scientists have been aware of a substance found in the serum of clotted blood which had the ability to cause powerful constriction of smooth muscle organs. Not until the mid-twentieth century did scientists at the Cleveland Clinic succeed in isolating this substance as a possible cause of high blood pressure. At the same time, investigators in Italy were busily trying to characterize the substance found in high concentrations in enterochromaffin cells of the intestinal mucosa. This material also had the ability to cause constriction of smooth muscular elements, particularly those of the gut. The material isolated from the bloodstream was given the name "serotonin" while that from the intestinal tract was called "enteramine." Subsequently, both materials were crystallized and shown to be identical with 5-hydroxytryptamine (5-HT) which could then be prepared synthetically, and shown to possess all the biological features of the natural substance. The indole nature of this molecule bore many resemblances to the psychedelic drug LSD and with which it could be shown to interact on smooth muscle preparations *in vitro*.

When 5-HT was first found within the mammalian central nervous system, the theory arose that various forms of mental illness could be due to biochemical abnormalities in its synthesis.

This line of thought was even further extended when the tranquilizing substance, reserpine, was observed to deplete brain 5-HT; throughout the duration of the depletion, profound behavioral depression was observed. As we shall see, many of these ideas and theories are still maintained although we have much more ample evidence now on which to evaluate them.

Occurrence

Indolealkyl amines (Fig. 6-1), including serotonin, occur widely in nature. For example, many types of fruits and vegetables such as pineapples and bananas contain extremely large amounts of 5-HT. In mammals, the highest concentration of this amine occurs in the pineal gland and in the enterochromaffin cells of the intestinal tract. In man, it is estimated that about 90 per cent of the body's serotonin occurs in the gastrointestinal tract,

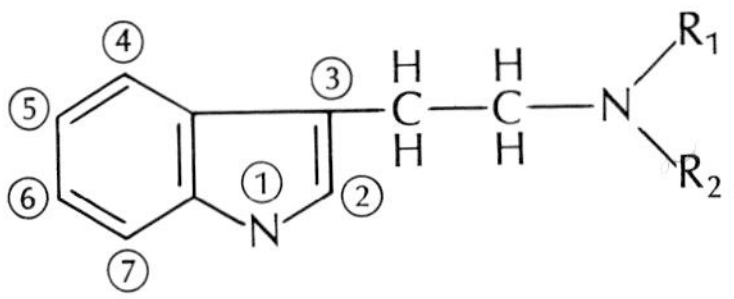

FIGURE 6-1. Structural relationships of the various indolealkylamines.

Molecule	Substitutions
Tryptamine	R_1 and $R_2 = H$
Serotonin	Tryptamine with 5 Hydroxy
Melatonin	5 methoxy, N—acetyl
DMT*	R_1 and $R_2 =$ methyl
DET*	R_1 and $R_2 =$ ethyl
Bufotenine*	5 hydroxy, DMT
Szara psychotrope*	6 hydroxy, DET
Psilocin*	4 hydroxy, DMT
Harmaline*	6 methoxy; R_1 forms isopropyl link to C_2.

* = psychotropic or behavioral effects.

another 8 to 10 per cent in platelets, and only 1 to 2 per cent within the central nervous system. In many of the laboratory animals, such as rats and mice, an additional tissue source of serotonin comes from the mast cell.

Chemical Properties and Assay

Serotonin is usually prepared as the creatinine sulfate salt with a solubility of approximately 20 mg/ml in water. The solution is stable at low pH but is easily oxidized in air, particularly above pH7. Serotonin is not soluble in alcohol, acetone, chloroform, or ether. Upon extraction from tissues, the more common methods for assay of serotonin are currently based on fluorescence spectrophotometry. Many of the early contradictory results in serotonin assay arose because the methods depended upon bioassays, which are extremely variable and difficult to reproduce from laboratory to laboratory. However, with the development of the fluorescence method by Udenfriend and his colleagues in the early 1950's it became possible to have a reproducible method for critically assaying serotonin levels with sensitivity as low as 80 ng/gram. With current methods of column extraction and chromatographic separation, it has been possible to have even more sensitive methods for serotonin assay.

Biosynthesis of Serotonin

While serotonin does occur naturally in brain, it does not enter the brain readily from the blood stream because of its solubility characteristics. Therefore, we must now inquire into the methods by which the brain is able to synthesize its own serotonin.

The first step appears to be the uptake of the amino acid tryptophan, which is the primary substrate for the synthesis. Plasma tryptophan arises primarily from the diet, and elimination of dietary tryptophan can profoundly lower the levels of brain serotonin. In addition, an active uptake process is known to facilitate the entry of tryptophan into cells, and this entry site can be

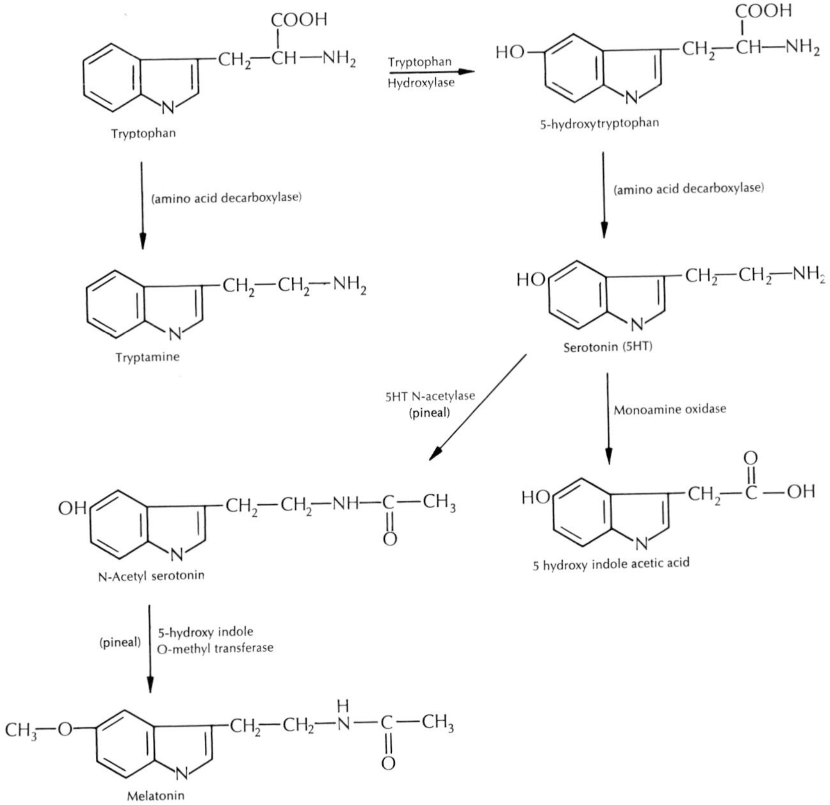

FIGURE 6-2. The metabolic pathways available for the synthesis and metabolism of serotonin.

competed for by certain other amino acids, such as phenylalanine. Because plasma tryptophan has a daily rhythmic variation in its concentration, it seems likely that this concentration variation could profoundly influence the rate and synthesis of brain serotonin.

The next step in the pathway to synthesize serotonin is to hydroxylate the molecule at the 5 position (Fig. 6-2) to form 5-hydroxytryptophan (5-HTP). The enzyme responsible for this reaction, tryptophan hydroxylase, occurs in low concentrations in most tissues, including the brain, and it was very difficult to isolate for study. However, by purifying the enzyme from mast cell tumors and determining the characteristic cofactors, it later became possible to characterize this enzyme in the brain. (Students should investigate the ingenious methods used for the initial assays of this extremely minute enzyme activity.) The enzyme as isolated from the brain appears to have an absolute requirement for molecular oxygen, reduced pteridine cofactor, and to require a sulfhydryl stabilizing substance, such as mercaptoethanol, for preservation of activity *in vitro*. With this fortified system of assay there is sufficient activity in the brain to synthesize one μg of 5-HTP per gram of brain stem in an hour. The pH maximum is approximately 7.2 and the K_m for tryptophan is 3×10^{-4}M. As it has been characterized thus far, tryptophan hydroxylase appears to be a soluble cytoplasmic enzyme; however, it must be remembered that the procedures used to extract it from the tissues may greatly alter the natural particle-binding situation.

This step in the synthesis can be specifically blocked by *p*-chlorophenylalanine, which competes directly with the tryptophan and also binds irreversibly to the enzyme. Therefore, recovery from tryptophan hydroxylase inhibition with *p*-chlorophenylalanine appears to require the synthesis of new enzyme molecules. In the rat, a single intraperitoneal injection of 300 mg/kg of this inhibitor lowers the brain serotonin content to less than 20 per cent within three days, and complete recovery does not occur for almost two weeks.

Decarboxylation

Following its synthesis, 5-HTP is almost immediately decarboxylated to yield serotonin. The enzyme responsible for this appears to be identical with the enzyme that decarboxylates dihydroxyphenylalanine (DOPA) (see Chapter 5). Since this de-carboxylation reaction occurs so rapidly, and since its K_m (5×10^{-6}M) requires less substrate than the preceding steps, trypto-phan hydroxylase would appear to be the rate-limiting step in the synthesis of serotonin, providing the added tryptophan is available in the controlled state. Because of this kinetic relation-ship, drug-induced inhibition of serotonin by interference with the decarboxylation step has never proven particularly effective.

Catabolism

For the most part, following its synthesis, the only effective route of continued metabolism for serotonin is to be deaminated by the enzyme monoamine oxidase. This enzyme is identical in all known characteristics with that which catabolizes the cate-cholamines. The product of this reaction, 5-hydroxyindoleacetal-dehyde can be further oxidized to 5-hydroxyindoleacetic acid (5-HIAA) or reduced to 5-hydroxytryptophol depending on the $NAD^+/NADH$ ratio in the tissue. Recently enzymes have been described in liver and brains by which 5-HT could be catabolized without deamination through formation of a 5-sulfate ester. This could then be transported out of brain, possibly by the acid ex-cretion system handling 5-HIAA.

Control of Serotonin Synthesis and Catabolism

Although there is a relatively brief sequence of synthetic and degradative steps involved in serotonin turnover, there is still much to be learned regarding the physiological mechanisms for controlling this pathway. At first glance, it seems clear that tryp-tophan hydroxylase is the rate-limiting enzyme in the synthesis of serotonin, since when this enzyme is inhibited by 80 per cent, the serotonin content of the brain rapidly decreases. On the other hand, when the 5-HTP decarboxylase is inhibited by equal or greater amounts, there is no effect upon the level of brain 5-HT. These data could only be explained if the important rate-limiting step were the initial hydroxylation. Since this step also depends upon molecular oxygen, the rate of 5-HT formation could also be influenced by the tissue level of oxygen. In fact, it can be shown that rats permitted to breathe 100 per cent oxygen greatly increase their synthesis of 5-HT. It is also of interest that 5-hydroxytryptophan does not inhibit the activity of tryptophan hydroxylase.

If the situation for serotonin were similar to that previously described for the catecholamines, we might also expect that the concentration of 5-HT itself could influence the levels of activity at the hydroxylation step. However, when the catabolism of 5-HT is blocked by monoamine oxidase inhibitors, the brain 5-HT concentration accumulates linearly to levels three times greater than controls, thus suggesting that end-product inhibition by serotonin is, at best, trivial. Similarly, if the efflux of 5-HIAA from the brain is blocked by the drug probenecid (which appears to block all forms of acidic transport) the 5-HIAA levels also continue to rise linearly for prolonged periods of time, again suggesting that the initial synthesis step is not affected by the levels of any of the subsequent metabolites. Two possibilities therefore remain open: the initial synthesis rate may be limited only by the access of required cofactors or substrate, such as oxygen, pteridine, and tryptophan from the bloodstream, or by other more subtle control features, more closely related to brain activity. Let us now consider the experiments which suggest that neuronal activity might influence the synthesis and metabolism of brain serotonin.

Pineal

The pineal organ is a tiny gland (1 mg or less in the rodent) contained within connective tissue extensions of the dorsal surface of the thalamus. While physically connected to the brain, the pineal is cytologically isolated for all intents, since it is on the "peripheral" side of the blood permeability barriers (see Chapter 2) and since its exclusive innervation arises from the superior cervical sympathetic ganglion. The pineal is of interest for two reasons. First, it contains all the enzymes required for the synthesis of serotonin, and two enzymes for subsequent use of the serotonin that are found in no other organs. In fact, the pineal contains more than fifty times as much 5-HT per gram as the whole brain. Second, the metabolic activity of the pineal 5-HT enzymes can be controlled by numerous external factors, including the neural activity of the sympathetic nervous system operating through release of norepinephrine. As such, the pineal appears to offer us a potential model for the study of brain 5-HT.

Actually, the 5-HT content of the pineal was discovered after the isolation of a pineal factor known to induce pigment lightening effects on skin cells. When this "melatonin" was crystallized and its chemical structure determined as 5-methoxy-N-acetyltryptamine, an indolealkylamine, a reasonable extension was to analyze the pineal for 5-HT itself. The production of melatonin from 5-HT requires two additional enzymatic steps. The first is the N-acetylation reaction to form N-acetylserotonin. This intermediate is the preferred substrate for the final step, the 5-hydroxy indole-O-methyl transferase reaction, requiring S-adenosyl methionine as the methyl donor.

The melatonin content, and its influence in suppressing the female gonads, was subsequently found to be enhanced by environmental light and suppressed by darkness. In fact, the established cyclic daily rhythm of both 5-HT and melatonin in the pineal appear to be directly related to environmental lighting patterns. Furthermore, this effect requires the presence of an intact sympathetic innervation, since chronically denervated pineal behaves biochemically like the pineal of a blinded animal. However, the controlling step by which the nerve impulses influence melatonin synthesis (and presumably the secretion from the pineal into the bloodstream) appears to be at the O-methylation step rather than earlier in the synthesis of 5-HT. Thus, the proposed model's applicability to brain 5-HT loses its lustre since this regulatory step does not seem to be of functional importance in the central nervous system. Furthermore, the "adrenergic" sympathetic nerves are now known to be able to take up 5-HT as well as they can take up and bind norepinephrine. Whether this is a functional mistake (to be able to secrete an endogenous false transmitter) or is simply a case of mistaken biologic identity, remains to be shown. It seems likely, however, that it is the neuronal norepinephrine whose release is required to pass on the intended communications from the sympathetic nervous system. The norepinephrine may cause its effects in the postjunctional cells by stimulating the synthesis of 3′, 5′ adenosine monophosphate (cyclic AMP) which in turn provides a controlling message to the sites synthesizing melatonin.

Localizing Brain Serotonin to Nerve Cells

While some of these pineal curiosities may prove to be useful for the study of brain 5-HT, they are no substitute for data derived directly from brain. If we attempt to relate changes in brain 5-HT and 5-HT metabolites to changes in brain activity with drug treatments or with different behavioral states, we must ascertain that brain serotonin is contained within nerve fibers. Although the brain content of serotonin was discovered in 1953, it was nearly ten years before scientists developed techniques which permitted us to know with certainty that the serotonin of the brain was contained in neurons. The first support for this view arose from studies on brain homogenates (see Chapter 3) in which it could be shown that the synaptosome fraction was rich in serotonin and 5-HTP-decarboxylase.

While this finding suggested only a general relationship to nerve terminals, two other techniques quickly appeared which related 5-HT to specific nerve tracts much more succinctly. A classical neuroanatomical approach has been to produce lesions and to follow the distribution of the degenerating axons. By combining this approach with biochemical measurements, Heller and Moore placed lesions in the medial forebrain bundle of the hypothalamus and observed that the forebrain concentration of serotonin dropped dramatically over the next 5 to 12 days (see Chapter 3). These data strongly suggested that a nerve pathway containing serotonin passed through the lateral hypothalamus; when the pathway was interrupted, degeneration of the axons resulted in loss of serotonin. At almost the same point in time, the Swedish histochemical group led by Hillarp and Falck, perfected the technique for using fluorescence histochemistry to reveal the distribution of monoamine-containing nerve fibers and cell bodies in the central nervous system. By this technique, almost all the serotonin-containing cell bodies were found to be restricted to a narrow group of neurons, known as the raphe nuclei, lying in the mid-portion of the lower pons and upper brain stem. Their fibers to the forebrain would follow the path predictable by the lesioning method of Heller and Moore. In many other laboratories, using different species of mammals, other investigators have established that by placing lesions at selected points along this postulated pathway from brain stem to forebrain or spinal cord, predictable drops of serotonin occur—provided the lesions are extensive enough to remove most of the raphe nuclei. However, very small lesions of individual portions of the raphe nuclei do not result in complete elimination of serotonin from any part of the rat's brain; this indicates that the raphe nuclei are likely to have extremely diffuse and presumably overlapping fields of innervation.

It would seem pertinent to attempt to localize the serotonin-containing nerves with electron microscopy. The numerous attempts to do so have concentrated mainly upon the cellular distribution and morphological characteristics of the nerve terminals arising from the raphe neurons. These nerve terminals can be identified in two ways. The easier way is to examine areas rich in the fluorescence labeling for serotonin nerve terminals; an alternative method is to attempt to label the endogeneous stores of serotonin by intraventricular injection of radioactive serotonin. The latter technique is based on the assumption that serotonin-containing neurons exhibit a specific uptake mechanism for their amine similar to that found in the catecholamine-containing neuron (see Chapter 5). After intraventricular injection of radioactive serotonin, the majority of the nerve terminals that are labeled exhibit large granular vesicles and numerous small electronlucent vesicles (Fig. 6-3). These nerve terminals are in a regional distribution which generally agrees with that described by fluores-

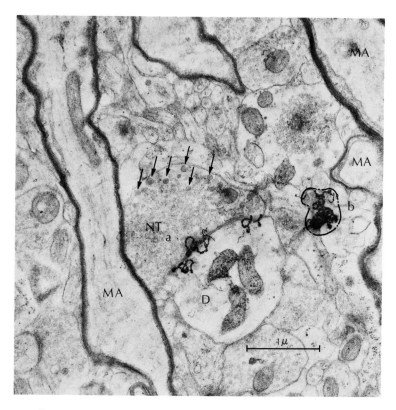

FIGURE 6-3. Low-power electron microscopic autoradiograph localizing radioactive serotonin in nerve terminals of the rat brain stem. The irregular silver coils can be seen along the zone of specialized contact over a nerve terminal (NTa), as well as over a small axon (b). Within the labeled nerve terminal (a) numerous large granular vesicles can be seen (arrows). Also visible in this field are other unlabeled nerve terminals and three myelinated axons (MA).

cence histochemistry. When brain slices from 5-HT-rich regions are incubated *in vitro* with a false marker, such as α-methyl norepinephrine, and then fixed with cold KMnO$_4$, nerve terminals in those portions of the brain which normally contain serotonin can be shown to exhibit small electron-dense synaptic vesicles just as those described for the norepinephrine-containing neurons. Furthermore, when lesions are made in the raphe nuclei, degenerative changes in these types of nerve endings can be found in the serotonin-rich neuropil of the suprachiasmatic nucleus. However, each of these methods is based on an indirect mechanism for revealing serotonin and no discrete specific histochemical technique with practical application to the central nervous system has yet been worked out.

CELLULAR EFFECT OF 5-HT

From the biochemical and morphological data above we can be relatively certain that the 5-HT of the brain occurs not only within the nerve cells but within specific tracts or projections of nerve cells. We must now inquire into the effects of serotonin when applied at the cellular level (see Chapter 2). In those brain areas in which microelectrophoretically administered 5-HT has been tested on cells which exhibit spontaneous electrical activity, the majority of nerve fibers are found to respond by decreasing their discharge rate. The effects observed typically last much longer than the duration of the microelectrophoretic current. However, in certain portions of the brain, particularly the limbic cortex, 5-HT can also be shown to cause pronounced activation of discharge rate. Since activation with 5-HT occurs much less commonly than depression with 5-HT, data are needed to verify that the activation response does not arise secondarily from inhibition of adjacent inhibitory interneurons.

However, in the simpler nervous system of molluscs, the application of serotonin can be shown to cause pronounced depolarization of cells being recorded with intracellular electrodes and there can be little question of the site of action. Rather convincing data on the vagal inhibitory reflex indicate that serotonin-containing interneurons may play an integral role in control of gastric contractions. If such is the case, then all other peripheral autonomic ganglia, in which serotonin content has been attributed to mast cells, will have to be reinvestigated.

In the mammalian central nervous system, however, we as yet have no specific synaptic connection which we can analyze for the effects of neurally released serotonin as compared with the effects of serotonin administered by micropipettes. Because of this acute lack of information, it is impossible to evaluate objectively the multiple reports in the literature concerning the specificity of alleged central serotonin blocking agents which affect neuronal and behavioral activity. Furthermore, practically no data exist on which we could predict whether or not such presumptive serotonin-mediated synapses are more likely to be excitatory or inhibitory or whether they are to control primary neurons or interneurons. This distinct lack of basic information should be borne in mind as we now review the cellular pharmacology and multicellular effects attributable to the serotonin system of the brain.

Cellular Pharmacology of Brain Serotonin

Let us first consider whether or not a dynamic re-uptake and turnover of serotonin occurs in a fashion similar to that described above for the catecholamines. If we attempt to use the same techniques, namely, to place a small amount of radioactive serotonin, into the ventricle to label the endogeneous stores of serotonin, and follow the decline in specific radioactivity of serotonin in the brain, we find that the serotonin half-life is very long, on the order of 4 to 5 hrs after the initial acute drop is over. When this ventricular labeling technique is verified by fluorescence histochemistry or light-microscopic or electron-microscopic autoradiography, the majority of the uptake is seen to be into those nerves that normally contain serotonin, but the labeling is mainly over terminals and axons with very little labeling within the cell body area. Therefore, we know, initially, that the labeling of the serotonin pool by these injection techniques is not complete and that the decline in radioactivity does not reflect total brain 5-HT. Furthermore, if we use any of the other methods for estimating turnover, such as inhibiting monoamine oxidase and following the rate of rise of serotonin, or inhibiting the efflux of 5-HIAA from the brain, we find that the biochemical estimate of this turnover is considerably faster than that determined by the labeling with radioactive 5-HT.

There would seem to be at least two explanations for this kinetic discrepancy. One would be that the uptake for serotonin is, in some respect, less selective or specific than that for the catecholamines. However, the uptake system appears to be similar in that it is energy dependent, that is, it is much more active at 37°C than at 0°, it requires both glucose and oxygen, and can be inhibited by ouabain, dinitrophenol, or iodoacetate. Furthermore, the uptake system for 5-HT can be partially inhibited by the same types of drugs which inhibit the uptake of catecholamine into catecholamine-containing nerve endings, such as desmethylimipramine, chlorpromazine, or cocaine, when evaluated on brain slices. When the nerve slices are stimulated, the serotonin previously taken up can be released into the media, suggesting—again—that the binding and release are by functional nerve fibers of a specific selective class.

On the other hand, when the turnover rates of brain serotonin (that is, complete whole brain serotonin) are estimated by using precursor labeling (i.e. tryptophan) and determining specific activity changes with time, results are mainly compatible with the fast rather than the slow turnover time of serotonin. The logical tentative conclusion to be reached then is that the pool of neuronal serotonin which the ventricular injection most readily labels consists mainly of the excess or storage form of serotonin, whereas total endogeneous serotonin, in terms of synthesis and utilization, is turned over much more rapidly. These findings would suggest that a great deal of serotonin resides in the storage form, patiently awaiting the call to action.

The Reserpine Story

One of the first drugs found empirically to be effective as a central tranquilizing agent, reserpine, was employed mainly for its action against hypertension. In the early 1950's when both brain serotonin and the central effects of reserpine were first described, there was great excitement when it was shown that the dramatic effects of reserpine upon the brain were to deplete the serotonin content. However, it shortly became clear that the norepinephrine and dopamine content of the brain could also be depleted by reserpine and that the depletion lasted longer than the sedative action. The brain levels would remain down for weeks while the acute behavioral effect was over within 48 to 72 hours. Hence, it became difficult to determine whether it was the loss of brain catecholamine or serotonin which accounted for the behavioral depression after reserpine. Perhaps in passing we should note the possibility that the behavioral effect and the biochemical effect might both be epi-phenomena of some more basic brain action.

Experiments were then performed which were mainly pseudo-behavioral in context, in which the reserpine-induced depression was combated by injecting heroic amounts of precursor amino acids, namely, 5-HTP or DOPA. When this is done, 5-HTP increased the sedation, but in even larger doses caused excitation. However, the recovery from reserpine-induced sedation was not typically related to the return of the brain serotonin level that resulted from the 5-HTP administration. On the other hand, when DOPA was injected (although the doses required are really quite large with respect to the amount of amine in the brain) the reserpine symptoms could be reversed. Furthermore, it was found that by treating with small doses of reserpine for long periods of time, one could deplete practically all of the brain catecholamines without causing behavioral symptoms, but when a subsequent large dose of reserpine was given and the norepinephrine content dropped an additional 10 per cent, the behavioral depression symptoms appeared.

All these experiments then were interpreted as favoring the view that depression after reserpine was mainly due to loss of brain catecholamines. However, we should note that the enzyme which catabolizes both these precursor amino acids is the same, and until it can be shown that the nerve terminals have the specific uptake mechanisms for the appropriate amino acid precursor but not the related amino acid, these findings alone do not necessarily give the correct answer to the reserpine problem.

More extensive experiments into the nature of this problem were possible when the drugs which specifically block the synthesis of catecholamines or serotonin were discovered. After depleting brain serotonin content with parachlorophenylalanine, which effectively removed 90 per cent of brain serotonin, investigators observed that no behavioral symptoms reminiscent of the reserpine syndrome appeared. Moreover, when p-chlorophenylalanine-treated rats, which were already devoid of measurable serotonin, were treated with reserpine, typical reserpine-induced sedation arose. These results again favor the view that loss of catecholamines could be responsible for the reserpine-induced syndrome. Furthermore, when α-methyl-p-tyrosine is given and synthesis of norepinephrine is blocked for prolonged periods of time, the animals are behaviorally sedated and their condition resembles the depression seen after reserpine. Therefore, after fifteen years of intensive work upon the possible cellular explanation for the behavioral action of reserpine, we are able to explain this action partially. The students will find it profitable to review in detail the original papers describing the results just summarized, and the other theories currently in vogue.

Hallucinogenic Drugs

One of the more alluring aspects of the study of brain serotonin is the possibility that it is this serotinergic system of neurons through which the hallucinogenic drugs cause their effects. In the early 1950's the concept arose that LSD might produce its behavioral effects in the brain by interfering with the action of serotonin there as it did in smooth muscle preparations, such as the rat uterus. However, this theory of LSD action was not supported by the finding that another serotonin blocking agent, 2-bromo LSD, produced minimal behavioral effects in the central nervous system. And, in fact, it was subsequently shown that very low concentrations of LSD itself—rather than blocking the serotonin action—could potentiate it. However, none of these data could be considered particularly pertinent since all the research was done on the peripheral nervous system and all the philosophy was applied to the central nervous system.

Shortly thereafter Freedman and Giarman initiated a profitable series of experiments investigating the basic biochemical changes in the rodent brain following injection of LSD. Although their initial studies required them to use bioassay for changes in serotonin, they were able to detect a small (on the order of 100 ng/g, or less) increase in the serotonin concentration of the rat brain shortly after the injection of very small doses of LSD. Subsequent studies have shown that a decrease in 5-HIAA accompanies the small rise in 5-HT. Although the biochemical effects are similar to those that would be seen from small doses of monoamine oxidase inhibitors, no direct monoamine oxidase inhibitory effect of LSD has been described. This effect was generally interpreted as indicating a temporary decrease in the rate at which serotonin was being broken down, and it could also be seen with higher doses of less effective psychoactive drugs. In related studies by Costa and his coworkers, who estimated the biochemical turnover of brain serotonin, prolonged infusion of somewhat larger doses of LSD clearly promoted a decrease in the turnover rate of brain serotonin.

The next advance in the explanation of the LSD response was made when Aghajanian and Sheard reported that electrical stimulation of the raphe nuclei would selectively increase the metabolism of 5-HT to 5-HIAA. This finding suggested that the electrical activity of the 5-HT cells could be directly reflected in the metabolic turnover of the amine. Subsequently, the same authors recorded single raphe neurons during parenteral administration of LSD and observed that they slowed down with a time course similar to the effect of LSD. Thus, following LSD administration both decreased electrical activity of these cells and decreased transmitter turnover occur. Two explanations for these events have been provided; one is that the LSD occupies serotonin receptor sites and thus activates some undefined feedback mechanism whereby the activity of the serotonin neurons is inhibited. On the other hand, the effects of LSD could be mediated by a direct inhibition of the serotonin-containing cells, either by a metabolic action or by blocking those neurotransmitters that normally activate these cells. Recently the latter point has been partially supported by data indicating that activation of raphe cells by either norepinephrine or 5-HT applied electrophoretically can be blocked by LSD.

Even though we can offer almost complete explanations for the biochemical parameters on 5-HT accompanying the effects of LSD, can we explain the behavioral responses to LSD in terms of these mechanisms? That is to say, if the effects of LSD as reflected in abnormalities of 5-HT metabolism were due primarily or exclusively to interactions with the raphe nuclei, then we should be able to reproduce the behavioral effects by other similar mechanisms. In light of the foregoing experiments, one might expect that removal of the raphe system would closely mimic the effects of LSD if the latter serves only to block 5-HT synapses. However, the physiological manipulation which most closely reproduces certain of the behavioral features of the LSD response, namely, failure to habituate to sensory stimuli, is best reproduced by electrical stimulation of the raphe nuclei. These data would suggest that at least a portion of the behavioral symptomatology requires the activation of the receptors opposite serotonin-containing nerve endings. There are other psychoactive drugs whose basic chemical structure is similar to that of serotonin (see Table 1). However, the majority of these compounds are much less active on a weight basis as compared with LSD, and explanation for their cellular mechanism of action will be even more difficult.

MULTICELLULAR BRAIN FUNCTIONS INVOLVING SEROTONIN

While we recognize that there is no single synaptic connection we can point to with certainty as being mediated by serotonin, there are, nevertheless, compelling data that serotonin-containing neurons are involved in certain multicellular functions of the brain.

Temperature Regulation

In the chick, cat, dog, and monkey, intraventricular injection of microgram quantities of serotonin will produce profound elevation of body temperature. An elevation of body temperature also follows electrical stimulation of the rat raphe nuclei; this latter effect can be prevented if serotonin is previously depleted by either reserpine or p-chlorophenylalanine. The increase in body temperature could either be due to stimulation of mechanisms which elevate temperature or to inhibition of mechanisms which are able to prevent hyperthermia. In this regard, treatment with p-chlorophenylalanine, while removing brain serotonin, does not in itself produce hypothermia. Thus, while these experiments suggest that 5-HT may play some role in temperature regulation, they do not explain whether the effects are central or peripheral or whether they are either species specific or brain-region specific.

Sensory Perception

We have already considered the possibilities that 5-HT may have some relationship to abnormal behavioral states such as those induced by tranquilizing or hallucinogenic drugs. In addition, animals treated with p-chlorophenylalanine were found to exhibit decreased motor activity, decreased emotional reactivity, and increased sensitivity to painful stimuli. The increased sensitivity to painful stimuli may be responsible for the observation that animals so treated are able to learn brightness discrimination more quickly since brightness discrimination is a somewhat painful stimulation; however, *p*-chlorophenylalanine treatment has no effect on the rate of learning of position discrimination.

When the raphe nuclei are stimulated electrically, animals fail to habituate to noise or repetitive sensory stimuli. This effect is similar to that seen during treatment with LSD as mentioned above. By whatever mechanism 5-HT-containing neurons are able to alter the perception or reaction to sensory stimuli, there apears to be a definite involvement, since blocking of serotonin synthesis also reduces the ability of rodents to become tolerant to chronic morphine injection.

Sleep

Several interrelated observations suggest that brain 5-HT is intimately involved in the mechanisms responsible for the various states of sleep. After either monoamine oxidase inhibition or intracerebral or intraventricular injection of 5-HT or 5-HTP, or after parenteral administration of 5-HTP there is electro-encephalographic evidence of increased time spent in slow-wave sleep. If brain serotonin content is drastically reduced either by electrical ablation of the raphe nuclei or by pretreatment with *p*-chlorophenylalanine, there also is a marked decrease in the amount of slow-wave sleep time. The relative loss of sleep time appears proportional to the extent of the serotonin loss. On the other hand, electrical stimulation of the raphe nuclei does not induce slow-wave sleep and one wonders what mechanisms are required in order for the serotonin cells to complete those brain mechanisms responsible for the onset of slow-wave sleep.

Furthermore, other brain amines appear relevant—at least pharmacologically—in sleep. Jouvet has suggested that the catecholamine and acetylcholine neuron participation may be most important in the transition from slow-wave sleep to rapid eyemovement sleep (also known as REM, paradoxical, or dream sleep). It has also been shown that gamma-hydroxybutyrate (see Chapter 7) and certain short chain fatty acids will also induce sleep when injected parenterally under the right conditions. Thus the multicellular mechanisms controlling sleep phases do not belong exclusively to the 5-HT system of neurons.

Summary

In this chapter we have encountered one of the more striking examples of an intensively studied brain biogenic amine for which there is every reason to believe that it is an important synaptic transmitter. Still to be determined are the precise synaptic connections at which this substance accomplishes the transmission of information and the functional role these connections play in the over-all operation of the brain with respect to both affective and other multicellular interneuronal operations. With the exception of *p*-chlorophenylalanine, the drug that blocks serotonin synthesis at the tryptophan hydroxylase step, the central pharmacology of serotonin is poorly elucidated, particularly with respect to drugs that are specific postsynaptic blocking agents. The study of brain serotonin appears likely to be a most fruitful area for future research in the field of neuropsychopharmacology.

Aghajanian, G. K., and D. X. Freedman (1968). Biochemical and morphological aspects of LSD pharmacology. In *Psychopharmacology—A Review of Progress* (D. H. Efron, ed.), pp. 1185. Government Printing Office, Washington, D.C.

Bloom, F. E. (1969). Serotonin neurons: Localization and possible physiological role. *Adv. Biochem. Psychopharmacol. 1*, 27.

Diaz, P. M., S. H. Ngai and E. Costa (1968). Factors modulating brain serotonin turnover. *Adv. Pharmacol., 75.*

Falck, B., N.-A. Hillarp, G. Thieme, and A. Torp (1962). Fluorescence of catecholamines and related compounds condensed with formaldehyde. *J. Histochem. Cytochem, 10*, 348.

Fuxe, K., T. Hokfelt, and U. Ungerstedt (1968). Localization of indolealkylamines in CNS. *Adv. Pharmacol. 6A*, 235.

Garattini, S., and L. Valzelli (1965). *Serotonin.* Elsevier Press, Amsterdam.

Garattini, S., P. A. Shore, E. Costa, and M. Sandler (1968). Biological role of indolealkylamine derivatives. *Adv. Pharmacol. 6A and 6B.*

Giarman, N. J., and D. X. Freedman (1965). Biochemical aspects of the actions of psychotomimetic drugs. *Pharmacol. Rev. 17*, 1.

Harvey, J. A., A. Heller, and R. Y. Moore (1963). The effect of unilateral and bilateral medial forebrain bundle lesions on brain serotonin. *J. Pharmacol. 140*, 103.

Jouvet, M. (1968). Neuropharmacology of sleep. In *Psychopharmacology, A Review of Progress.* D. Effron, editor, Government Printing Office, Washington, D.C., p. 523.

Neff, N. H., R. C. Lin, S. H. Ngai, and E. Costa (1969). Turnover rate measurements of brain serotonin in unanesthetized rats. *Adv. Biochem. Psychopharmacol. 1*, 91.

Wurtman, R. J., J. Axelrod, and D. E. Kelly (1968). *The Pineal,* Academic Press, New York.

7 | γ-Aminobutyric Acid, Glycine, and Glutamic Acid

Synthesised in 1883, γ-aminobutyric acid (GABA) was known for many years as a product of microbial and plant metabolism. Not until 1950, however, did investigators identify GABA as a normal constituent of the mammalian central nervous system and find that no other mammalian tissue, with the exception of the retina, contains more than a mere trace of this material. Obviously, it was thought, a substance with such an unusual distribution must have some characteristic and unique phyisological effects which might make it important for the function of the central nervous system. Almost twenty years later we still have no conclusive proof as to the role this compound plays in the mammalian central nervous system, although much evidence has accumulated supporting the hypothesis that it is an inhibitory transmitter.

Distribution

In mammals, GABA has been detected in brain and spinal cord but not in peripheral nerve tissue such as sciatic nerve, splenic nerve, sympathetic ganglia, or in any other peripheral tissue such as liver, spleen, or heart. These findings give some idea of the uniqueness of the occurrence of GABA in the mammalian central nervous system. Like the monoamines, GABA also appears to have a discrete distribution within the central nervous system. However, unlike the monoamines, the concentration of GABA found in the central nervous system is in the order of μmoles/gm rather than nmoles/gm. It is interesting that brain also contains large amounts of glutamic acid (8-13 μmoles/gm), which is the main source of GABA. In the rat, the corpora quadrigemina and the diencephalic regions contain the highest levels of GABA, while much lower concentrations are found in whole cerebral hemispheres, the pons, and medulla; white matter contains relatively low concentrations of GABA. Recently, the discrete localization of GABA in the brain of anesthetized monkeys has been determined by Fahn and Côté and by DeFeudis *et al.* Some of this data is summarized in Table 7-1. It should be noted that endogenous levels of GABA increase rapidly post mortem: a 30 to 45 per cent increase in GABA occurs within two minutes after death in the rat if the tissue is not instantly frozen *in situ.* The origin of this sudden increase is unknown, but it seems quite unlikely that it could be solely explained by *de novo* synthesis.

Progressive increases in GABA levels and in glutamic acid decarboxylase activity appear to occur in various regions of the brain during development. The high levels of GABA found in the various regions of the brain of the Rhesus monkey appear to correlate well with the activity of glutamate decarboxylase, the enzyme responsible for the conversion of L-glutamate to GABA. This is not the case for the degradative enzyme GABA-transaminase, since the globus pallidus and the substantia nigra, which have the highest concentration of GABA, have a relatively low transaminase activity. There also does not appear to be a consistent inverse relationship between GABA concentration and transaminase activity. Thus, some areas of brain, such as the dentate nucleus and the inferior colliculus, which have relatively high concentrations of GABA also have large amounts of transaminase activity.

TABLE 7-1. Regional Distribution of GABA in Monkey Brain

	Region of brain	n	μmoles/g frozen tissue $\pm$ S.E.M.
Highest	substantia nigra	4	9.70 $\pm$ 0.63
	globus pallidus	4	9.54 $\pm$ 0.91
	hypothalamus	4	6.19 $\pm$ 0.13
High	inferior colliculus	4	4.70 $\pm$ 0.29
	dentate nucleus	3	4.30 $\pm$ 0.47
	superior colliculus	3	4.19 $\pm$ 1.09
	periaqueductal gray	3	4.02 $\pm$ 0.56
Medium	putamen	4	3.62 $\pm$ 0.21
	pontine tegmentum	4	3.34 $\pm$ 0.43
	caudate nucleus	4	3.20 $\pm$ 0.18
	medial thalamus	4	3.00 $\pm$ 0.14
Low	lateral thalamus	4	2.68 $\pm$ 0.09
	occipital cortex	4	2.68 $\pm$ 0.23
	anterior thalamus	4	2.50 $\pm$ 0.23
	medullary tegmentum	4	2.27 $\pm$ 0.22
	inferior olivary nucleus	4	2.25 $\pm$ 0.15
	frontal cortex	4	2.10 $\pm$ 0.01
	motor cortex	4	2.09 $\pm$ 0.10
	cerebellar cortex (not pure gray)	4	2.03 $\pm$ 0.23
Lowest	centrum semiovale (pure white)	4	0.31 $\pm$ 1.0

Data taken from: Fahn, S., and Côté, L. J. (1968).

Since GABA does not easily penetrate the blood-brain barrier, it is difficult if not impossible to increase the brain concentrations of GABA by peripheral administration, unless one alters the blood-brain barrier. Some investigators have tried to circumvent this problem by the administration of GABA-lactam (2-pyrrolidinone) to animals in the hope that this less polar and more lipid soluble compound would penetrate more easily into the brain and be hydrolyzed to yield GABA. Although the idea seems plausible, it does not succeed: the GABA-lactam that reaches the central nervous system is not hydrolyzed to any extent.

Metabolism

There are three primary enzymes involved in the metabolism of GABA prior to its entry into the Krebs cycle. The relative activity of enzymes involved in the degradation of GABA suggest that, similar to monoamines, they play only a minor role in the termination of the action of any neurally released GABA.

Figure 7-1 outlines the metabolism of GABA and its relationship to the Krebs cycle and carbohydrate metabolism. As mentioned previously, GABA is formed by the α-decarboxylation of L-glutamic acid, a reaction catalyzed by glutamic acid decarboxylase, an enzyme which occurs uniquely in the mammalian central nervous system and retinal tissue. The precursor of GABA, L-glutamic acid can be formed from α-oxoglutarate by transam-

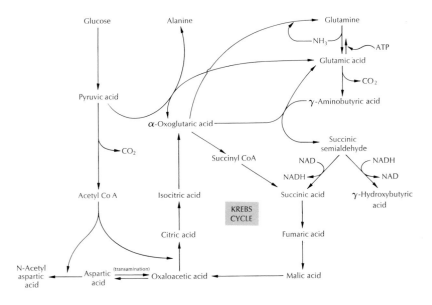

FIGURE 7-1. Interrelationship between γ-aminobutyric acid and carbohydrate metabolism.

ination or reaction with ammonia. GABA is intimately related to the oxidative metabolism of carbohydrates in the central nervous system by means of a "shunt" involving its production from glutamate, its transamination with α-oxoglutarate by GABA-α-oxoglutarate transaminase (GABA-T) yielding succinic semialdehyde and regenerating glutamate, and its entry into the Krebs cycle as succinic acid via the oxidation of succinic semialdehyde by succinic semialdehyde dehydrogenase. In essence then the "shunt" bypasses the normal oxidative metabolism involving the enzymes α-oxoglutarate dehydrogenase and succinyl thiokinase.

From a metabolic standpoint, the significance of the "shunt" is unknown; energetically at least it is less efficient than direct oxidation through the Krebs cycle (3 ATP equivalents versus 3 ATP + 1 GTP for the Krebs cycle). Experimentally, it has been quite difficult to make an adequate assessment of the quantitative significance of the "shunt" in the oxidation of α-oxoglutarate *in vivo*. Studies with ^{14}C-labeled glucose both *in vivo* and *in vitro* have indicated that the carbon chain of GABA can be derived from glucose. Therefore, in some cases the incorporation of radioactivity into the "shunt" metabolites following the injection of uniformly labeled ^{14}C-glucose has been used to assess the functional aspects of this "shunt." However, these experiments are somewhat inconclusive since they do not necessarily indicate the rate of flux through this pathway. Some relatively indirect experiments have given results suggesting that about 10 to 40 per cent of the total brain metabolism may funnel through this "shunt."

Glutamic Acid Decarboxylase (GAD)

GAD is the enzyme responsible for the conversion of L-glutamic acid to GABA. It appears to be the only enzymatic pathway for GABA formation in the brain, and the decarboxylation goes virtually to completion. No reversal of this reaction has been demonstrable either *in vivo* or *in vitro*. In mammalian organisms this relatively specific decarboxylase is found only in the central nervous system, where it occurs in higher concentrations in the gray matter. In general, the localization of this enzyme in mammalian brain correlates quite well with the GABA content. So far this enzyme has been purified about 200-fold from mouse brain. It has a pH optimum of about 6.5, requires pyridoxal phosphate, and is inhibited by various anions. This inhibition by anions may be interesting from a physiological standpoint. The possibility has been raised that variations in the chloride concentration at a given nerve ending could control GABA formation. Although there is no evidence of wide variations in chloride content under normal physiological conditions, it is of interest that in snail brain the D cells (depolarized by acetylcholine) and the H cells (hyperpolarized by acetylcholine) have different chloride contents. In fact, the D cells have an internal chloride content about three times that of the H cells. The GAD isolated and purified from lobster inhibitory nerve is inhibited by concentrations of GABA (0.1 M) similar to the actual endogenous concentrations found in the inhibitory fiber. This raises the possibility that GABA may control its own formation via product inhibition of GAD. Potassium ion and β-mercaptoethanol are essential for activity of the purified lobster enzyme.

GABA-Transaminase (GABA-T)

GABA-T, unlike the decarboxylase, has a wide tissue distribution. Therefore, although GABA cannot be formed outside the central nervous system, exogenous GABA can be rapidly metabolized by both central and peripheral tissue. However, since endogenous GABA has not been detected in cerebrospinal fluid or blood it is unlikely that it ever leaves the brain intact. The brain transaminase has a pH optimum of 8.2 and also requires pyridoxal phosphate. It appears that the coenzyme is more tightly bound to this enzyme than it is to GAD. The brain ratio of GABA-T/GAD activity is almost always greater than one. Sulfhydryl reagents tend to decrease GABA-T activity, suggesting that this enzyme requires the integrity of one or more sulfhydryl groups for optimal activity. The transamination of GABA catalyzed by GABA-T is a reversible reaction, so if a metabolic source of succinic semialdehyde were made available it would be theoretically possible to form GABA by the reversal of this reaction. However, as indicated below, this does not appear to be the case *in vivo* in normal or experimental conditions so far investigated.

Recent studies with more sophisticated cell fractionation techniques and electron microscopic monitoring of the fractions obtained have borne out the original claims that both GAD and GABA-T are particulate to some extent. GAD was found associated with the synaptosome fraction, whereas the GABA-T was largely associated with mitochondria. Further studies on the mitochondrial distribution of GABA-T have suggested that the mitochondria released from synaptosomes have less activity than the crude unpurified mitochondrial fraction, and it has been inferred that the mitochondria within nerve endings have little GABA-T activity. This finding has led to the speculation that GABA is metabolized largely at extraneuronal intercellular sites or in the postsynaptic neurons.

Succinic Semialdehyde Dehydrogenase (SSADH)

Brain succinic semialdehyde dehydrogenase (SSADH) has a high substrate specificity and can be distinguished from the nonspecific aldehyde dehydrogenase found in brain. The enzyme purified from human brain has a pH optimum of about 9.2 and quite a low Michaelis constant (K_m) for succinic semialdehyde of 5.3×10^{-6}. SSADH from rat brain has a similarly low K_m for succinic semialdehyde of 7.8×10^{-5} and for NAD of 5×10^{-5}. The high activity of this enzyme and the low Michaelis constant, which allow the enzyme to function effectively at low substrate concentrations, probably account for the fact that succinic semialdehyde (SSA) has not even been detected as an endogenous metabolite in neural tissue despite the active metabolism of GABA *in vivo*. In contrast to SSADH isolated from bacterial sources where NADP is several times more active as a cofactor than NAD, the enzyme from monkey and human brain demonstrates a specificity for NAD as a cofactor. The regional distribution of this enzyme has been studied in human brain and found to parallel the distribution of GABA-T activity, although the dehydrogenase is about 1.5 times as active. The greatest activity was found in the hypothalamus, basal ganglia, cortical gray matter, and mesencephalic tegmentum. SSADH also has a marked heat activation at 38°C, and Pitts suggested that its activity *in vivo* might be regulated by temperature such that fever might result in an increased flux through the GABA shunt. This appears unlikely, however, since this step is usually not considered to be rate limiting in the conversion of GABA to succinic acid, and thus small changes in its activity would not be reflected in an over-all change in GABA metabolism. A sensitive and specific assay for SSADH is based on the fluorescence of NADH formed in the conversion of succinic semialdehyde to succinic acid. This method is sensitive enough to assay samples as small as 0.05 μg of freeze-dried brain tissue.

Since GABA's rise to popularity, the literature has been inundated with reports purporting to demonstrate that many pharmacological and physiological effects can be ascribed to and correlated well with changes in the brain levels of this substance. Since both GAD and GABA-T are dependent on the coenzyme pyridoxal phosphate it is not surprising that pharmacological agents or pathological conditions affecting this coenzyme can cause alterations in the GABA content of the brain. Epileptiform seizure can be produced by a lack of this coenzyme or by its inactivation. Conditions of this sort also lead to a reduction in GABA levels, since GAD appears to be preferentially inhibited over the transaminase, presumably due to the fact that GAD has a lower affinity for the coenzyme than does GABA-T. A diet deficient in vitamin B6 in infants can lead to seizures that respond successfully to treatment consisting of addition of pyridoxine to the diet. However, it must be remembered that many other enzymes, including some of those involved in the biosynthesis of other bioactive substances, are also pyridoxal-dependent enzymes. A number of observations, in fact, indicate that there is no simple correlation between GABA content and convulsive activity. Administration of a variety of hydrazides to animals has uniformly resulted in the production of repetitive seizures following a rather prolonged latent period. The finding that the hydrazide-induced seizures could be prevented by parenteral administration of various forms of vitamin B_6 led to the suggestion that some enzyme system requiring pyridoxal phosphate as a coenzyme was being inhibited and that the decrease in the activity of this enzyme was somehow related to the production of the seizures observed. At this time attention focused on GABA and GAD because of their unique occurrence in the central nervous system and because GAD had been shown to be inhibited by carbonyl trapping agents *in vitro*. The hydrazide-induced seizures were accompanied by substantial decreases in the levels of GABA and reductions in GAD activity in various areas of the brain studied. (This decrease in GABA produced by thiosemicarbazide is now believed to be due to a decrease in the rapid post-mortem increase in GABA mentioned previously.) The direct demonstration of the reversal of the action of the convulsant hydrazides by GABA itself proved to be difficult, due to the lack of ability of GABA to pass the blood-brain barrier in adult mammalian organisms. However, a preferential inhibition of GABA-T could be achieved *in vivo* with carbonyl reagents such as hydroxylamine (NH_2OH) or aminooxyacetic acid which resulted in an increase in GABA levels (up to 500 per cent of control) in the central nervous system. However, although these agents caused a decrease in the susceptibility to the seizures induced by some agents, such as metrazole, they did not exert any protective effect against the hydrazide-induced convulsions, even though they prevented the depletion of GABA and in some cases even increased the GABA levels above the controls. In fact, administration of very high doses of only aminooxyacetic acid instead of producing the normally observed sedation caused some seizure activity in spite of the extremely high brain levels of GABA.

An interesting finding with aminooxyacetic acid is that administration of this compound to a strain of genetically spastic mice in a single dose of 5-15 mg/kg results in a marked improvement of their symptomology for 12 to 24 hours. This improvement is associated with an increase in GABA levels, but the GABA level increases with a similar time course and to the same extent as in normal control mice. All studies to date indicate that the principal genetic defect in these mice is not in the operation of the GABA system. However, the drug-induced increase in GABA may serve to quell an excess of or imbalance in excitatory input in some unknown area of the central nervous system.

Hydrazinopropionic acid has recently been described as a potent inhibitor of GABA-T. It has been suggested that this compound inhibits GABA-T because of its close similarity to GABA with respect to structural configuration, molecular size, and molecular charge distribution. Its inhibitory action cannot be reversed by the addition of pyridoxal phosphate. Hydrazinopropionic acid is about 1000 times more potent than aminooxyacetic acid in inhibiting mouse brain transaminase.

Alternate Metabolic Pathways

In addition to undergoing transamination and subsequently entering the Krebs cycle, GABA can apparently undergo various other transformations in the central nervous system, forming a number of compounds whose importance, and in some cases natural occurrence, has not been conclusively established. Figure 7-2 depicts a variety of derivatives for which GABA may serve as a precursor. Perhaps the simplest of these metabolic conversions is the reduction of succinic semialdehyde (a product of GABA transamination) to γ-hydroxybutyrate (GHB). The transformation of GABA to GHB has been demonstrated in rat brain both *in vivo* and *in vitro*. In addition, the natural occurrence of GHB has been established by means of gas chromatography. Rat brain contains about 2 nmoles/gm while guinea pig brain contains almost twice this concentration. Among brain metabolites γ-hydroxybutyrate is rather unique in that this compound possesses anesthetic properties. Whether or not this compound

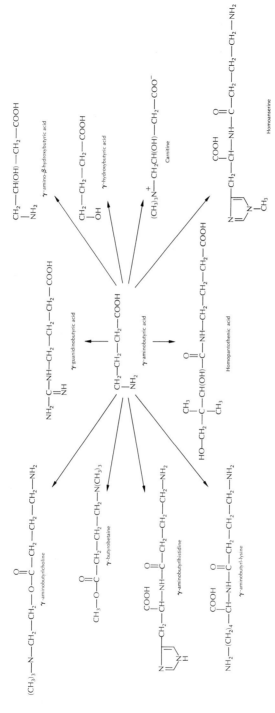

FIGURE 7-2. Possible alternate metabolic pathways for γ-aminobutyric acid.

plays any role in the normal sleep processes or in the pathogenesis of sleep disorders remains to be determined. GHB also has an interesting interrelationship with the catecholamines in that exogenously administered GHB or γ-butyrolactone (GBL) in doses which produce "sleep" (i.e. loss of righting reflex) causes a large increase in brain dopamine content with little or no effect on brain norepinephrine, serotonin, or GABA. This increase in brain dopamine induced by GHB appears to be largely a result of a decreased release or utilization of dopamine.

Several conflicting reports concerning the natural occurrence of γ-amino-β-hydroxybutyric acid (GABOB) in mammalian brain have appeared in the literature. Some investigators claim that GABOB occurs in mammalian brain in concentrations as high as four μmoles per gram. Others have reported its presence in much smaller amounts or its total absence. The most careful studies employing automated amino acid analysis and two-dimensional paper chromotography have indicated that GABOB is either absent in rat brain or present in amounts less than 0.01 μmoles per gram. However, despite the fact that little or no GABOB is present in brain, many electrophysiological investigations have been conducted to determine its possible action as a neuro-inhibitory substance. This compound has been claimed by some to block experimentally induced convulsions in animals when administered topically to the brain or even systemically. Also some investigators have claimed that GABOB is effective clinically in preventing and alleviating epileptic seizures. When administered iontophoretically to single neurons in the cerebral cortex, GABOB exerts a depressant effect comparable in potency to GABA. On the crayfish stretch receptor neuron, GABOB is only about one-half as potent as GABA.

γ-Aminobutyrocholine was detected in 1958 by paper chromatography in mammalian brain. More recently, a more rigorous identification has been made by Kewitz, who estimated the concentration in rat brain to be about 80 nmoles/gm. This choline ester appears to be resistant to hydrolysis by acetylcholinesterase while butyrocholinesterase has some limited capacity to hydrolize this substance at a rather slow rate. In addition, this ester does not appear to undergo transamination with α-oxoglutarate as does the parent compound—GABA. Although it produces a potent and prolonged depressant effect on the neuromuscular junction, its effects on the central nervous system have not been extensively studied. When the action of γ-aminobutyrylcholine was studied by means of iontophoresis onto cerebral cortical neurons there was relatively little depressant activity. In fact, the action was less than that of γ-aminobutyrobetaine, which is itself only a weak depressant. Curiously, when γ-aminobutyrylcholine was applied topically to the cerebral cortex its depressant potency was similar to that of GABA. In fact it is about 1000 times as active as GABA in suppressing metrazole-induced spikes in the EEG recording of the mammalian cortex. It has both a depressant and an excitatory action on Renshaw cells in the spinal cord.

γ-Butyrobetaine is a substance which has been known for many years to be present in tissues obtained from snakes and eels but only recently has it been suggested to occur in mammalian tissue. This compound has been only tentatively identified in the mammalian central nervous system in a complex with coenzyme A. Pharmacologically, the action of γ-butyrobetaine resembles to some extent that of acetylcholine, except that it is substantially less potent and has a more prolonged action on tissues such as the superior cervical ganglion, ileum, and the neuromuscular junction. γ-Butyrobetaine is pharmacologically inactive when iontophoresed onto cortical neurons.

γ-Guanidinobutyric acid also appears to be a normal metabolite of mammalian brain and could act as a source of GABA by means of transamidination. This compound can inhibit the crayfish stretch receptor but is somewhat less potent than GABA in this respect. A few drops of a 1 per cent solution applied topically markedly augments the evoked potentials of the cerebral cortex while it depresses the cerebellar response.

γ-Aminobutyrylhistidine (homocarnosine) has been reported to occur in beef brain (10-25 $\mu g/gm$), dog and cat brain (1.2

μg/gm), human brain (80 μg/gm), and frog brain (240 μg/gm), but the biological significance of this compound remains unknown.

Acetylcarnitine and carnitine have also been suggested to be normal metabolites of mammalian brain, although their occurrence is by no means restricted to this tissue. The esters of carnitine possess acetylcholine-like activity in a number of biological preparations.

It is not surprising that γ-aminobutyryl-lysine has recently been identified as a normal constituent of the rabbit central nervous system, since earlier studies had indicated that the enzyme which catalyzes the synthesis of carnosine and homocarnosine also forms peptides of GABA and various basic amino acids. However, although this compound seems to occur exclusively in the central nervous system, it does not appear to have any discrete regional localization. Degradation of this peptide appears to be catalyzed by a different enzyme than carnosinase, which usually attacks peptides containing an imidazole in the terminal carboxyl position. An enzyme catalyzing the degradation of γ-aminobutyryl-lysine and other peptides with arginine, lysine, and ornithine in their carboxyl terminals has been found in brain.

Neurotransmitter Role

Quite a strong case can be made for a transmitter role for GABA at inhibitory nerve endings to the muscle or to stretch receptor neurons in crustacea. The evidence can be summarized as follows:

1. Externally applied GABA duplicates the effects of inhibitory nerve stimulation at the crustacean neuromuscular junction as well as at other crustacean synapses.
2. Both exogenous GABA and the endogenous inhibitory transmitter substance when in contact with postsynaptic membrane or receptor site cause this membrane to become more permeable to chloride ion. This increase in chloride permeability in both cases can be blocked by picrotoxin.

3. GABA appears to be the most potent inhibitory compound extractable from the lobster nervous system.
4. Inhibitory axons and cell bodies in the lobster nervous system have a much higher content of GABA than excitatory axons or cell bodies, the GABA ratio found being on the order of 100 : 1. The endogenous GABA content of the inhibitory axon is approximately 0.1M.
5. The enzymes necessary for the formation and destruction of GABA are present in the inhibitory axon and cell body.
6. A specific GABA uptake mechanism, which could be involved in transmitter inactivation, analogous to the norepinephrine system, has been described in the crayfish stretch receptor and the lobster nerve-muscle preparation. However, it is not known if the uptake is primarily into presynaptic nerve terminals.
7. Most recently it has been demonstrated that GABA is released by the lobster nerve-muscle preparation during stimulation of the inhibitory axons. This release was shown to be frequency dependent. Moreover, stimulation of the excitatory nerve to the same muscle does not liberate GABA. Also, GABA release induced by stimulation of the inhibitory fibers can be blocked by lowering the Ca^{++} content of the medium, which also blocks neuromuscular transmission.

Neurotransmitter Role in the Mammalian Central Nervous System

The action of GABA in the crustacean nervous system has sometimes been used as indirect evidence that this substance also functions as a neurotransmitter in the mammalian central nervous system. While there is no doubt that these speculations have served to generate a great deal of interest, the observations made in the crustacean nervous system cannot substitute for data on the events taking place in the mammalian nervous system.

The evidence from the central nervous system to support a

role of GABA as an inhibitory transmitter is still somewhat deficient. With substances such as the amino acids, which may play a dual role (both in metabolism and as neurotransmitters), it is only to be expected that it will be more difficult to obtain conclusive evidence as to their role as neurotransmitters. The elementary criteria for identification of a compound as a putative transmitter have already been mentioned. In short, the agent in question must be produced, stored, released, exert its appropriate action, and be removed from its site of action. There is sufficient evidence for the production, storage, and pharmacological activity of GABA consistent with its suggestive role as an inhibitory transmitter, but it has not yet been possible to demonstrate an association of GABA with specific inhibitory pathways in the cortex. Until recently there was also no evidence that GABA could be released from mammalian brain under physiological conditions. Several reports now claim to have demonstrated the spontaneous release of GABA from the surface of the brain. However, only one group of investigators has claimed that the amount of GABA released from the cortex is dependent upon the activity of the brain. This group has found that in cats showing an aroused EEG, either following cervical cord section or in awake animals receiving local anesthesia, small amounts of GABA will leak out of the cerebral cortex and can be recovered by a superfusion technique (cortical cup) provided the pia-arachnoid membrane has been punctured. This release of GABA into cortical cups occurs about three times more rapidly from the brains of cats showing an EEG sleep-like pattern with marked spindle activity following midbrain section than in cats showing an EEG awake pattern. When a continuous waking state was maintained by periodic stimulation of the brain stem reticular formation, no measurable amounts of GABA could be found in the perfusates. Investigators have reported difficulty in repeating these observations, perhaps due to a rapid uptake of GABA back into the cortex. However, DeFeudis, Delgado, and Roth have been able to demonstrate the release of newly synthesized GABA (and other amino acids) from deep brain nuclei of monkeys such as

FIGURE 7-3. Amino acid profile and semi-logarithmic plots of the distribution of radioactivity after perfusion of the right caudate nucleus of a Rhesus monkey with ^{14}C-glucose. A volume of 2.28 ml was collected every minute and a 1.5 ml aliquot was counted for radioactivity; 29 mg of caudate nucleus and its corresponding perfusate collected over ½ hr (0.5 ml) were analyzed. Buffer changes and elution time are indicated. Since the column of resin used for the perfusate was 2 cm shorter than that used for the extract, GABA was eluted sooner in this analysis but coincided exactly with the ninhydrin positive peak. Abbreviations: MSO, methionine sulfoxide; ASP, aspartate; GLN, glutamine; ASPN, asparagine; SER, serine; GLU, glutamate; PRO, proline; GLY, glycine; ALA, α-alanine; VAL, valine; ILE, isoleucine; LEU, leucine, TYR, tyrosine, PHE, phenylalanine; GABA, γ-aminobutyric acid. (Unpublished photograph, data in DeFeudis, Delgado, and Roth, 1970.)

---

the amygdala and caudate nucleus, using push-pull cannulas. As yet, this release has not been correlated with brain activity.

Figure 7-3 illustrates an automated amino acid analysis of an extract from a caudate nucleus perfused with uniformly labeled ^{14}C-glucose and the perfusate obtained from this structure. This technique has the advantage that it provides a rigorous establishment of the identity of the amino acids collected as well as enabling the detection of very minute amounts of these substances.

When GABA is applied iontophoretically to Deiters' neurons it induces IPSP-like changes and therefore mimics the action of the inhibitory transmitter released from axon terminals of the Purkinje cells. GABA is also known to be concentrated in Purkinje cells which exert a monosynaptic inhibitory effect on neurons of Deiters' nucleus. Very recently Obata and Takeda observed that stimulation of the cerebellum, which presumably activates the Purkinje cell axons, which have their terminals in cerebellar subcortical nuclei adjacent to the fourth ventricle, induces about a threefold increase in the amount of GABA released into the ventricular perfusate. However, the extremely

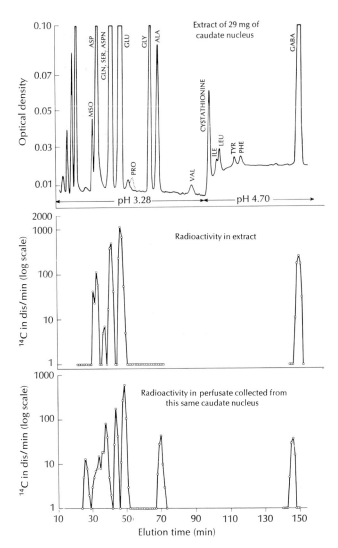

high voltage employed, the relatively crude perfusion system, and the lack of critical identification of GABA make the significance of these otherwise interesting observations on release somewhat questionable, although they are consistent with the hypothesis that GABA is an inhibitory transmitter in the particular pathway.

In addition, other recent experiments have indicated that labeled GABA can be released from brain slices by electrical stimulation or by the addition of high potassium to the incubation medium. However, one should bear in mind that all the above-mentioned release experiments are somewhat gross in nature and do not provide evidence with regard to the neuronal system involved in the release of GABA or even if this release is in any way associated with an inhibitory synaptic event. In fact, at the present time no suitable test system in the CNS has been developed which will be as appropriate as the lobster nerve-muscle preparation. The student is advised against holding his intellectual breath until it has.

Most of the investigations analyzing the mechanism of GABA's depressive action on the central nervous system have been conducted on spinal cord motor neurons. Until quite recently GABA had not shown much evidence of closely mimicking the inhibitory transmitter. In fact, only a few years ago Curtis and his associates discounted the hypothesis that GABA might be the main inhibitory transmitter in the mammalian central nervous system. They noted that the action of GABA iontophoresed onto spinal neurons differed significantly from that of the inhibitory transmitter; whereas natural postsynaptic inhibition was associated with membrane hyperpolarization, experiments with coaxial pipettes failed to detect any hyperpolarization of motor neurons during the administration of GABA. Since at that time there was no evidence that GABA had a hyperpolarizing action in other parts of the central nervous system, Curtis concluded that GABA could not be the main central inhibitory transmitter. Recently, other investigators have demonstrated that in the cortical neurons of the cat GABA imitates the action of the cortical inhibitory transmitter at least qualitatively; it usually raises the membrane potential and increases conductance of cortical neurons, just like the normal inhibitory synaptic mechanism. When the latter inhibitory effect is artificially reversed by the administration of chloride into the neuron, the action of GABA is also reversed in a similar way. Similar results have been obtained on neurons in Deiters' nucleus. Therefore, at least as far as the cortex and Deiters' nucleus are concerned, there appears to be much support for the hypothesis that GABA is an inhibitory transmitter. Furthermore, the "negative data" obtained previously by Curtis have been criticized on conceptual and technical grounds.

There appears to be no pharmacologically sensitive mechanism for the rapid destruction of GABA similar to the cholinesterase mechanism for destruction of acetylcholine. Thus aminooxyacetic acid or hydroxylamine given intravenously or iontophoresed does not appear to prolong significantly the duration of action of iontophoretically applied GABA. The exception is Deiters' nucleus, where the hyperpolarization produced by GABA on the neurons in Deiters' nucleus and the IPSP are prolonged in both cases by hydroxylamine, an agent of dubious pharmacological specificity. No functional re-uptake mechanism for GABA within a mammalian system has been conclusively demonstrated either. However, GABA is actively and efficiently taken up by brain slices and this implies that some uptake phenomena are functional in the intact brain for recycling GABA and terminating its action. This mechanism could also explain why it has been difficult to collect GABA released from neural tissue. Unfortunately, no drug has been discovered which will block the uptake of GABA into nervous tissue without exerting a number of other unwanted pharmacological actions. One possible fruitful area of approach is to look for a specific inhibitor of GAD so GABA could be depleted selectively from the central nervous system. At present no really specific inhibitors for GAD have been developed that can inhibit this enzyme *in vivo* without also inhibiting GABA-T and a variety of other B_6-dependent enzymes. Another real advance would be the development of a histochemical method for the visualization of GABA at the electron microscope level. Equally important for the study of this system would be the specific drugs to block receptor sites.

So far it has been difficult to determine if any physiological or even pharmacological alteration of animal behavior produces alterations in the function of the GABA system in the intact animal. This is primarily because a simple and reliable technique has not been developed for the measurement of GABA turnover *in vivo*. Thus we are limited to looking at changes in the brain levels of GABA in order to glean some evidence concerning the activity of this system. Since the brain undoubtedly has many homeostatic mechanisms for the maintenance of GABA levels under widely varying conditions of activity, it would seem that changes in the activity of the GABA system, at least within the physiological range, would not necessarily lead to substantial changes in GABA concentration within the brain. Thus, development of any technique which could reliably evaluate the turnover of GABA *in vivo* would undoubtedly add to a better understanding of the functional importance of GABA in the central nervous system.

GLYCINE

As an Inhibitory Transmitter

Some evidence now exists which indicates that glycine may play a role as an inhibitory transmitter in the mammalian spinal cord. From the evidence available we will try to assess how well this compound fulfills the criteria necessary to categorize this substance as a central nervous system inhibitory transmitter. First, we can say that this amino acid is found in relatively high concentrations in the spinal cord compared with other amino acids. Table 7-2 illustrates the occurrence of glycine and other free amino acids in the spinal cord, and from these data it is apparent that glycine is more concentrated in the spinal gray matter than in the spinal white matter. The concentration found in the spinal gray matter is much higher than the level in whole brain or spinal roots. This high level of glycine in the ventral horn, together with the comparatively low content in ventral root fibers, initially suggested that glycine may be associated with the inhibitory interneurons, and subsequently this was shown to be the case. From iontophoretic studies the compounds in Table 7-2 can be divided into four main groups.

TABLE 7-2. Amino Acid Concentration of Cat Spinal Cord
and Roots ($\mu moles/g$)

Amino acids	Spinal gray	Dorsal root	Ventral root
Alanine	0.62	0.36	0.30
Arginine	0.14	0.07	0.06
Aspartate	2.14	0.79	1.13
Cystathionine	3.02	0.02	0.01
GABA	0.84	Trace	Trace
Glutamate	4.48	3.33	2.09
Glutamine	5.48	1.46	1.10
Glycine	4.47	0.28	0.32
Leucine	0.16	0.06	0.05
Lysine	0.16	0.07	0.05
Methyl-histamine	—	—	—
Serine	0.41	0.32	0.23
Threonine	0.21	0.18	0.15

Data taken from: M. H. Aprison and R. Werman (1968).

1. Excitatory — glutamate, aspartate
2. Inhibitory — GABA, glycine, alanine, cystathionine, and serine
3. Inactive — glutamine, leucine, threonine, and lysine
4. Untested — arginine and methyl histidine

Of the amino acids in group two, cystathionine and serine appear to have a weaker and relatively sluggish action on spinal neurons compared with that of GABA and glycine. Therefore, in view of the distribution and the relative inhibitory potency of the compounds in this group, it was suggested by Aprison and Werman that GABA and glycine were the most likely candidates for spinal inhibitory transmitters. Glycine administered by iontophoretic techniques was consistently found to diminish the firing and excitability of both spinal motor neurons and interneurons. This is interesting in itself since glycine is quite ineffective as an inhibitor of cortical neurons. In addition, the hyperpolarization and the changes in membrane permeability produced by glycine seem to be quite similar to those produced by the spinal inhibitory transmitter. Alteration in K^+ or Cl^- ion concentrations affect the inhibitory postsynaptic potentials and the glycine-induced potentials in the same fashion. Strychnine, a compound which has been shown to reduce spinal postsynaptic inhibition, also blocks the effects of glycine on spinal motor neurons. It was originally reported that strychnine reversibly blocks the action of the natural inhibitory synaptic transmitter(s), glycine and of β-alanine, but does not have any effect on the hyperpolarizing action of GABA in cats anesthetized with pentobarbital. However, similar experiments on decerebrated unanesthetized cats have indicated that the qualitative dichotomy between glycine and β-alanine and GABA originally reported does not usually hold. Instead, only a quantitative difference in the interaction of strychnine and the amino acids above is reported. In all these experiments, strychnine more potently antagonized glycine than GABA. However, GABA also inhibits these spinal neurons and is present endogenously, and in the course of distinguishing between the relative merits of GABA and glycine as inhibitory transmitter candidates in the spinal cord it was of interest to see if a loss of function of inhibitory interneurons would be accompanied by a change in one or both of these compounds. Anoxia of the lumbosacral cord produced by clamping the thoracic aorta seems to destroy the interneurons preferentially, while leaving 80 per cent or more of the motoneurons intact. Thus, the presynaptic cells responsible for inhibition (and other functions) are lost and therefore the concentration of transmitter associated with these cells would be expected to be decreased. When the effect of anoxia on GABA and glycine content of the cat spinal cord was analyzed, glycine was the only potential inhibitory amino acid markedly decreased. Thus the distribution of glycine in the spinal cord of the cat appears to be related to the inhibitory interneurons. In summary, glycine thus satisfies many of the criteria sufficiently to warrant its consideration as a possible inhibitory transmitter in the cat spinal cord.

    a. it occurs in the cat spinal cord associated with interneurons;

    b. when administered iontophoretically it hyperpolarizes motoneurons to the same equilibrium potential as post-synaptic inhibition;

    c. the permeability changes of the postsynaptic membrane induced by glycine appear to be similar to those associated with postsynaptic inhibition;

    d. strychnine, a drug which blocks the action of glycine, also blocks postsynaptic inhibition.

The mechanisms by which the action of iontophoretically applied glycine or that of the putative spinal inhibitory transmitters are terminated is not known at this time. Recently, it has been demonstrated that there is an active and efficient sodium-dependent uptake mechanism for glycine in rat spinal cord. However, whether or not this is the physiological mechanism by which the action of administered or released glycine is terminated remains to be determined. Also, to date very little appears to be known with regard to the release of glycine from the spinal cord. Again, as with GABA the efficient uptake process may explain why it is difficult to detect glycine release from the central nervous system. The main problem (as with GABA, glutamate, etc.) is that there is no distinct neuronal pathway which may be isolated and stimulated; thus all the induced activity is very generalized, making the significance of any demonstrable release (metabolite or excess transmitter) very difficult to interpret.

GLUTAMIC ACID

Both glutamic acid and aspartic acid are excitant amino acids found in significant quantities in the mammalian central nervous system. Thus, if any amino acid is involved in regulation of nerve cell activity, as excitatory synaptic transmitter or otherwise, it seems unnecessary, at least at present, to look beyond these two. However, we cannot yet say conclusively whether these substances are in fact transmitters in the central nervous system of mammals or, for that matter, even in invertebrates. In fact, the case for glutamate as a transmitter in the mammalian central nervous system is considerably weaker than that for acetylcholine, catecholamines, 5-HT, GABA, and glycine. In the vertebrate central nervous system, iontophoretic application of both glutamate and aspartate to nerve cells does produce depolarization and an increase in firing rate. In this connection, as was mentioned above, both GABA and L-glutamate are released from the cerebral cortex of the cat at a rate which appears to be dependent upon its state of activation—more GABA and less L-glutamic acid being released under conditions associated with "sleep-like" EEG patterns, with the reverse situation occurring under arousal conditions. This differential release does not appear to result from alterations in cortical blood flow, since the release of other amino acids such as L-glutamine and L-aspartic acid does not vary similarly with different conditions. However, at this time it was not demonstrated that the origin of these amino acids collected was in fact from neurons or, for that matter, even from brain cells. The possibility could not be ruled out that these amino acids were derived from blood or cerebrospinal fluid. Although these experiments can be taken as supportive evidence for a role of these agents as transmitters, they by no means establish this role.

Some disturbing facts are that glutamate, aspartate, and synthetic derivatives of these dicarboxylic acids result in almost universal activation of unit discharge, and they appear to be almost ubiquitous in the nervous system without the expected asymmetric distribution. It has also been reported that glutamate does not bring the cell membrane potential to the same level as the natural excitatory transmitter. In addition, both the D and L isomers are active, although in the case of glutamate the D isomer is often reported to be somewhat less active. These findings have led many investigators to suggest that the response to amino acids represents a nonspecific receptivity of the neuron to these agents and is therefore not indicative of a transmitter function. However, the possibility still exists that glutamate may serve as a final excitatory agent in the chemical events involved in synaptic transmission.

Aprison, M. H., and R. Werman (1968). A combined neurochemical and neurophysiological approach to identification of central nervous system transmitters. In: *Neurosciences Research*, Vol. 1, 157, Academic Press, New York.

Curtis, D. R., and J. M. Crawford (1969). Central synaptic transmission—microelectropheretic studies. *Ann. Rev. Pharmacol. 9*, 209.

Curtis, D. R., and J. C. Watkins (1965). The pharmacology of amino acids related to gamma-aminobutyric acid. *Pharmacol. Rev. 17*, 347.

De Feudis, F. V., J. M. R. Delgado, and R. H. Roth (1970). Content, synthesis and collectability of amino acids in various structures of brain of Rhesus monkeys. *Brain Research, 18*, 15.

Elliot, K. A. C. (1965). Aminobutyric acid and other inhibitory substances. *Brit. Med. Bull. 21*, 70.

Euler, C. von, S. Skoglund, and U. Söderberg (Eds.) (1968). *Structure and Function of Inhibitory Neuronal Mechanisms*. Pergamon, New York.

Fahn, S., and L. J. Cote (1968). Regional distribution of γ-aminobutyric acid (GABA) in brain of the Rhesus monkey. *J. Neurochem. 15*, 209.

Jasper, H. H., R. T. Kahn, and K. A. C. Elliott, (1965). Amino acids released from cerebral cortex in relation to its state of activation. *Science 147*, 1448.

Kewitz, H. (1962). Gamma-aminobutyrlcholine in the central nervous system. In: *Proc. First International Pharmacological Meeting*, Vol. 8, Pergamon, New York.

Obata, K. and K. Takeda (1969). Release of γ-aminobutyric acid into the fourth ventricle induced by stimulation of the cat's cerebellum. *J. Neurochem. 16*, 1043.

Quarton, G. C., T. Melnechuk, and F. O. Schmitt (1967). *The Neurosciences: A Study Program.* Rockefeller University Press, New York.

Roberts, E., C. F. Baxter, A. Van Harrefeld, C. A. G. Wiersma, W. R. Adey, and K. F. Killam (1960). *Inhibition in the Nervous System and Gamma-aminobutyric Acid*, Permagon, New York.

Roberts, E., and J. Kuriyama (1968). Biochemical-physiological correlations in studies of the γ-aminobutyric acid system. *Brain Res.* *8*, 1.

Roth, R. H., and N. J. Giarman (1970). Natural occurrence of gamma-hydroxybutyrate in mammalian brain. *Biochem. Pharmacol. 19*, 1087.

8 | Histamine, Prostaglandins, Substance P, Ergothioneine, and Cyclic AMP

HISTAMINE

A QUICK glance at this book reveals that the major emphasis on the biogenic amines in the nervous system has been devoted to norepinephrine, dopamine, and 5-hydroxytryptamine rather than histamine. This is due, in part, to the great bulk of contradictory evidence on histamine, especially regarding its possible relation to mental disease. Of course, some of the more recent conflicts may be resolved in view of the fact that the spectrophotometric assay so often used to measure brain histamine has been found to be completely unreliable since it measures other normal constituents of brain such as spermidine and histidine. Thus much of the research concerned with histamine in the central nervous system will have to be repeated with new methodology before it can be properly evaluated.

The actual physiological significance of brain histamine still remains obscure, even though its presence in nervous tissue has been recognized for many years. Certain peripheral nerves such as the sympathetic postganglionic fibers are particularly rich in histamine. Histamine is present in the hypothalamic and hypophyseal regions of the mammalian central nervous system. Its release from certain peripheral nerves implies a role for histamine as a transmitter substance, but the fact that the histamine content of sensory nerves usually rises progressively after degeneration, rather than being lost from the nerve like other putative transmitter substances, contradicts this implication.

In the hope of obtaining a better insight into the neuronal function of histamine, many studies have been carried out on the effect of exogenous histamine on transmission in the superior cervical ganglion of the cat. It is now known that small doses (as little as 0.1 μg) of histamine facilitate submaximal ganglionic transmission and potentiate the response of the ganglion to ACh, nicotine, carbachol, choline, and other substances. Histamine in higher doses (greater than 1 μg) directly stimulates the nonperfused ganglion, while the perfused ganglion is less sensitive to histamine. This effect is opposed by cocaine, morphine, and various depolarizing ganglionic blocking agents. Even larger amounts of histamine ($\sim$ 150 μg) block transmission of supramaximal preganglionic impulses through the superior cervical ganglion. These findings on the superior cervical ganglia are thus consistent with the hypothesis that histamine may function in the nervous system in a "neuromodulatory role." It is interesting that small amounts of histamine (1-4 μg) inhibit transcallosally evoked potentials in the cat cortex, suggesting that histamine may function as a synaptic inhibitor. Many workers in this field question the validity and significance of this finding since almost every agent tried in this system seems to produce inhibition. Applied iontophoretically to neurons in the lateral geniculate and spinal cord, histamine has little or no activity. On cortical neurons, however, histamine has some inhibitory effects although it is much less potent than γ-aminobutyric acid.

The large quantities of histamine (up to 100 μg/gm, seven times that of the adrenergic transmitter) in postganglionic sympathetic fibers also suggests that it may participate in some way in the regulation of peripheral nervous activity. However, little evidence for the existence of histaminergic nerves has been forth-coming over the years. In fact, the histamine in these nerves has often been ascribed to mast cells and has been considered to be un-related to axons. Yet the histamine found in mast cell granules sediments with material denser than mitochondria, while the par-ticulate histamine in splenic nerve sediments with material of less density than mitochondria. In addition, it has been observed that perfusion of the sciatic nerve with compound 48/80, a substance which releases mast cell histamine, only released about 25 per cent of the nerve histamine. *In vivo* treatment of dogs with either 48/80 or reserpine does not deplete postganglionic sympathetic nerves of histamine. These experiments support the contention that the histamine in these nerves is not associated with mast cells.

Mast cells are absent from the central nervous system, except for restricted areas, and the histamine there must reside in some other cellular component. The subcellular distribution of brain histamine is consistent with the hypothesis that it is contained in nerve endings. It is also of interest that the general pattern of dis-tribution of histamine in the brain is much like that of the other biogenic amines such as norepinephrine and 5-hydroxytrypta-mine. The concentration is high in the hypothalamus (in fact there is twice as much histamine as 5-hydroxytryptamine here), intermediate in the midbrain, and lowest in the cortex and white matter. It is surprising that many investigators refer to the 0.1-0.5 μg/gm of histamine found by Crossland and Garven as very low and therefore of doubtful significance. Yet it is commonly stated that the hypothalamus contains a high concentration of 5-hydroxy-tryptamine, although its actual content is often no more than about 0.5 μg/gm.

Recent experiments have shown that cat brain can form his-tamine from histidine and can convert histamine to methyl histamine and methylimidazole acetic acid (Fig. 8-1). The meth-ylating enzyme imidazole-*N*-methyltransferase has been iso-lated from cat brain. For many years it was believed that the en-zyme responsible for the formation of histamine from histidine was the nonspecific aromatic-L-amino acid decarboxylase. The properties of this enzyme have been described in some detail in Chapter 5. However, recent experiments have uncovered a rather specific histidine decarboxylase existing in various mammalian

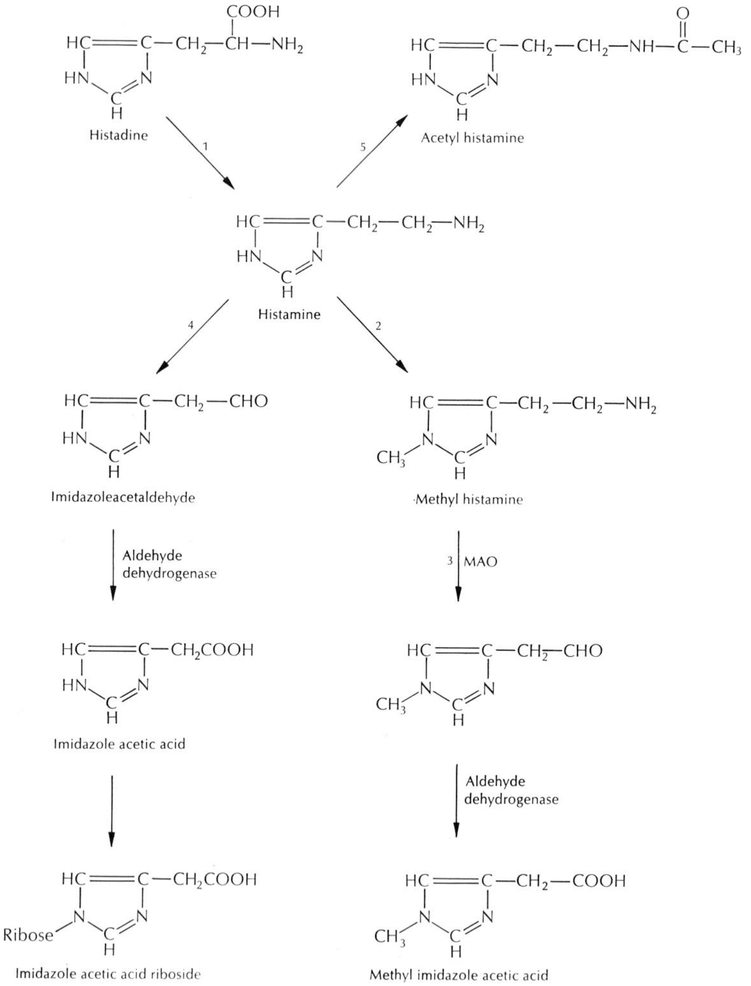

FIGURE 8-1. Metabolism of histamine. (1) Histidine decarboxylase. (2) Histamine methyl transferase. The major pathway for inactivation in most mammalian species. (3) Monoamine oxidase. (4) Histaminase. (5) Minor pathway of histamine catabolism.

tissues. Whether or not this specific enzyme is the enzyme responsible for the formation of histamine in neuronal tissue has yet to be conclusively demonstrated. A prototype for the specific histidine decarboxylase has been partially purified from fetal rat tissue. This enzyme is inhibited by α-methylhistamine but not to any extent by α-methylDOPA, an inhibitor of aromatic amino acid decarboxylase.

Histamine metabolism in the brain is influenced by drugs known to be centrally active. Reserpine, for example, reduces the concentration of histamine in the hypothalamus and thalamus just as it reduces the concentration of other amines there, although not to the same extent. Tremorine also decreases brain histamine. Chlorpromazine, which partially inhibits N-methyltransferase, increases the histamine concentration. However, these findings give little insight into the function of histamine in the central nervous system. Unlike other bioactive amines, histamine is not taken up against a concentration gradient by brain slices.

PROSTAGLANDINS

In 1935 Euler discovered a substance in human seminal plasma and sheep vesicular glands which he thought was secreted by the prostate gland. This substance, for which he coined the name "prostaglandin," appeared to be an active acidic lipid with smooth muscle stimulating and depressor activity. Since the chemical structure of this class of substances was not elucidated until almost thirty years later, the term "prostaglandin"—although a misnomer—had sufficient time to become firmly ingrained in the literature. In fact, this term is still used today as a generic name for the whole class of chemical compounds, occurring naturally in a variety of tissues, all of which are related derivatives of prostanoic acid. Thus, the term "prostaglandin" is now generically applied to designate one of sixteen or more chemically distinct natural constituents extractable from various mammalian tissues. There are two major series of prostaglandins, the E series in which the five-membered ring has one hydroxyl and one keto

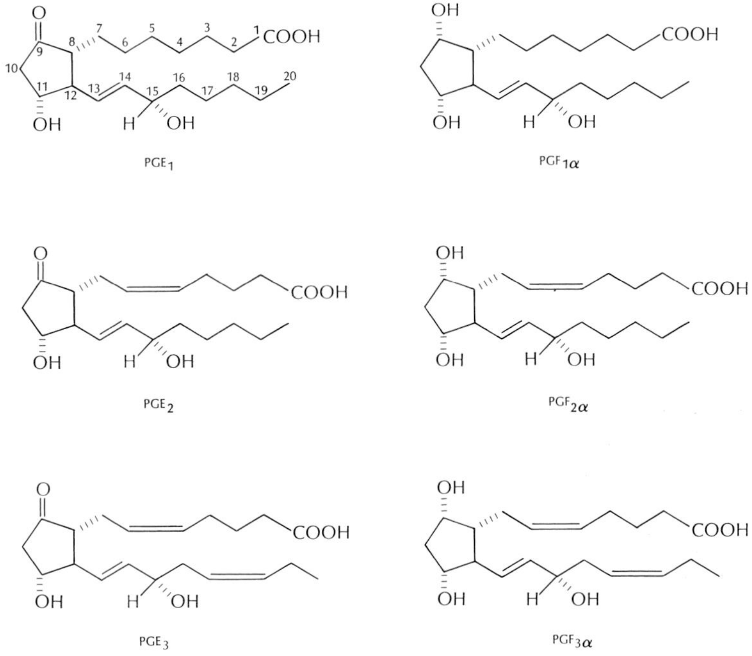

FIGURE 8-2. Structure of prostaglandins.

group and the F series in which the substituents are both hydroxyls (Fig. 8-2). Although many different biological roles have been ascribed to or postulated for this class of compounds, we will limit our discussion here to their postulated role as neurotransmitters or neuromodulators.

In numerous peripheral tissues the release of prostaglandins has been shown to be associated with nerve activity. The release of prostaglandins from the stomach can be induced by vagal or transmural stimulation. However, it has been claimed that this release is from muscle cells and not from nerve terminals since stomach strips stored in the cold for three days to allow degeneration of nerve fibers still release prostaglandins. Stimulation of the splenic nerve in dogs and cats also causes an output of large amounts of prostaglandin E_2 (PGE_2) (200 ng/ml) in the venous effluent. Pretreatment of the spleen with an α-adrenergic blocking agent such as phenoxybenzamine or phentolamine abolishes both the splenic contraction and the output of prostaglandins in response to nerve stimulation or catecholamine injection. PGE₁ perfused through the spleen does not cause splenic contraction and therefore the action of PGE as a neurotransmitter in this preparation can be ruled out since it does not mimic the effects of nerve stimulation. However, PGE may play a modulatory role on sympathetic neuroeffector systems. This seems quite likely in the spleen since the administration of PGE diminishes the contractile response of the spleen to nerve stimulation and also decreases the nerve induced output of norepinephrine. It thus seems likely that at many peripheral sites prostaglandins are not even putative transmitters, since the released prostaglandins do not usually mimic the effects of nerve stimulation.

It is now quite well established that the central nervous system contains a number of different prostaglandins. In addition, these substances are also normal constituents of cerebrospinal fluid. Generally, the mammalian CNS contains predominantly the PGF$_\alpha$ series with small amounts of a PGE in some cases. The concentration of prostaglandins found in the mammalian central nervous system is in the range of 100-200 ng/gm. There are also a few reports indicating that brain has the enzymatic capacity for the synthesis of some prostaglandins. The current view is that PGE's are stored minimally and most of that released from the brain derives from a newly synthesized pool. The distribution of these substances in the central nervous system appears to be fairly uniform and certainly does not vary widely enough to suggest that prostaglandins may be exclusively associated with specific pathways in the brain as are the many other putative transmitters already considered in previous chapters.

The various prostaglandins can produce potent effects on the central nervous system. Thus, the injection of 7-20 μg/kg of PGE into the cerebral ventricles of cats produces catatonia and somnolence, whereas PGF$_{2\alpha}$ in similar doses is without effect. In young chicks, where the blood-brain barrier is not fully developed, intravenous PGE₁ produces profound sedation. In addition

PGE_1 and $PGF_{2\alpha}$ appear to have direct actions on spinal neurons. Thus PGE administered intravenously or applied topically to the cord causes an increased excitability of α motoneurons. When prostaglandins are iontophoresed onto single neurons in the cortex they are found to be without observable effects. On the other hand prostaglandins iontophoresed onto spontaneously firing neurons in the medulla and caudal pontine region of the cat central nervous system produced either an increase, decrease, or no change in the firing rate. Recent experiments also demonstrate that both PGE_1 and PGE_2 have specific effects in blocking norepinephrine depression of rat cerebellar Purkinje cells. However, so far it has not been determined whether in fact any of the prostaglandins mimic the action of the natural inhibitory or excitatory transmitters at central synaptic sites.

Many prostaglandins are released from superfused cat cerebral or cerebellar cortex. The release from the somatosensory cortex can be greatly increased by direct or contralateral stimulation of the cortex. If the corpus callosum is sectioned, the release is limited to the stimulated side. Release from the cortex can also be increased by afferent nerve stimulation. The release induced in the contralateral cortex by stimulation of the radial nerve is frequency dependent, being maximal at 0.25-1/sec and minimal at 30-100/sec. Prostaglandin release has also been demonstrated in ventricular perfusates. Again, although much research has been devoted to the release of prostaglandins from central sites, it has not been possible to determine the release of prostaglandins from localized areas of the central nervous system in response to stimulation of well-defined anatomical pathways in the central nervous system. A number of pharmacological stimulants can also evoke the release of prostaglandins from the central nervous system. The most notable are picrotoxin, pentylenetetrazole, and strychnine.

Studies on rat brain cortical homogenates indicate that PGE may be to some extent associated with the synaptosome fraction, although not with synaptic vesicles. The biosynthetic enzymes appear, however, to be localized to the microsomal fraction.

None of the above evidence is indicative of prostaglandins acting as typical central nervous system neurotransmitters. However, four lines of evidence indirectly support a role for the prostaglandins in transmission processes within the central nervous system.

1. They are found as natural constituents of the mammalian central nervous system and can be synthesized by the brain.
2. They are released from the brain and spinal cord and this release can be increased by direct or indirect stimulation of the brain.
3. Certain prostaglandins have potent—albeit gross—pharmacological actions on the central nervous system when administered intraventricularly or to species with underdeveloped blood-brain barrier.
4. PGE_1 appears to be concentrated in the synaptosome fraction isolated from rat brain.

SUBSTANCE P

In 1931 Euler and Gaddum were assaying ACh in extracts from brain and intestine when they detected the presence of another pharmacologically active substance, later named substance P because it was isolated in the form of a powder. This name has turned out to be much more appropriate than the authors realized some 35 years ago since it is now known that substance P is in fact structurally a polypeptide. However, to date its physiological function is still quite obscure. The only difference in the substance P of intestinal origin and that isolated from the central nervous system appears to be the greater lability of the brain preparation. Pharmacologically, this substance has both smooth muscle contractile activity and vasodilatory activity. In these pharmacological actions substance P is one of the most potent agents known, especially on a molar basis, since 2 to 3 ng injected into man will produce a marked effect on blood flow. Throughout the many years following its discovery there have been numerous reports concerning the central nervous system effects produced by this substance. However, the highly purified preparation of Haefely and Hürlimann lacks any significant effect on the central nervous system even when administered in high doses intravenously or intracerebrally, so it must be concluded that the pharmacological effects reported originally were due largely to impurities in the preparation.

More recently the properties of increasingly purer (1-2×10^5 times the potency of the original preparation of Euler and Gaddum) preparations of substance P have been more fully investigated. Most of the purest preparations contain a basic polypeptide composed of the same 13 amino acids. The molecular weight of this peptide has been estimated to be about 1000. One of the greatest difficulties in preparing and purifying this material is that it becomes more and more unstable with each stage of purification.

Substance P is distributed almost exclusively in the digestive tract and the nervous system. All peripheral nerves and ganglia studied appear to contain this substance, and it is found in all the layers of the intestine. Euler observed that substance P is present in peripheral nerves in subcellular particles (microsomes) from which it can be released by hypotonic solutions, acid, or heat treatment. However, no evidence is available to suggest whether or not substance P is stored in similar subcellular particles in brain. All determinations of the distribution of substance P in the central nervous system of cats, dogs, cattle, and humans have been made by bioassay. The more recent quantitative estimations have been made by means of the terminal ileum of the guinea pig. The assays are usually performed in the presence of atropine, a serotonin antagonist, and an antihistamine, in order to prevent the stimulant effect on the gut of acetylcholine, 5-hydroxytryptamine, and histamine, any or all of which could occur in tissue extracts. These precautions do not necessarily exclude the possibility that materials other than substance P are acting on the ileum, but the presence of another polypeptide (bradykinin) can be excluded by using the hen's rectal caecum, which is either insensitive or relaxes in the presence of bradykinin. Even despite the difficulty in accurately bioassaying this material, there appears to be general agreement that this substance is widely distributed in nervous tissue, with a localized distribution in certain parts of the brain. In general, the concentration of substance P appears to decrease with increasing differentiation of the central nervous system. In human brain the substantia nigra contains the highest concentration, approximately 1000 units/gm. Next in order are the floor of the fourth ventricle and the inferior colliculus, followed by the midbrain, hypothalamus, caudate nucleus, and thalamus. With the exception of the spinal cord, white matter contains less substance P than gray matter. In the spinal cord there is an interesting discrepancy between dorsal and ventral roots. The dorsal roots contain about ten times as much substance P as the ventral roots.

This unequal distribution in various brain regions together with the finding that brain contains an enzyme that inactivates substance P has led some investigators to postulate a transmitter role for this substance. However, at this time there is very little evidence to support such a conclusion. The enzymes responsible for the synthesis of substance P are unknown and have therefore not been localized. While there is no direct evidence that substance P is released during neuronal activation, retinal substance P increases in animals maintained in darkness and decreases after exposure to light, implying that the levels within this tissue may be controlled by impulse activity. Most importantly, substance P has not been demonstrated to produce any effects on individual neurons. Only two positive bits of evidence favor a functional role for this substance: the report that the concentration of substance P decreases in degenerating neurons, and the report that during Wallerian degeneration of sensory nerves the concentration of substance P in the proximal stump increases while that in the distal end falls This functional interpretation may be strengthened by the observation that since substance P has not been detected in glial cell tumors it may therefore be localized in nerve cells. This would seem to be a rather poor foundation for any self-respecting transmitter candidate.

ERGOTHIONEINE

Although the cerebellum is richly endowed with nervous connections to other areas of the brain, it appears to be surprisingly lacking in pharmacologically active substances (acetylcholine, norepinephrine, dopamine, and 5-hydroxytryptamine) which are found in abundance elsewhere in the CNS. The knowledge of this high density of neurons and synaptic connections coupled with the apparent lack of recognizable bioactive substances was no doubt the impetus which stimulated Crossland's interest in examining this structure for other pharmacologically active substances. Cerebellar extracts possessed a factor which increased the electrical activity of the cerebellum when injected into the cerebral circulation. This factor is stable in alkali and unstable in acid, and although exhibiting activity on central neurons, it is inactive on smooth or striated muscle or autonomic ganglia. The active principle of this factor has recently been tentatively identified as ergothioneine (the betaine of thiolhistidine, see Fig. 8-3), although there is some controversy as to its identification. Both the cerebellum and the optic nerve have relatively high concentrations of this substance (4.9 and 28.7 μg/gm respectively). However, its action at cerebellar synapses remains unknown. A careful investigation of the actions of this substance on the cerebellum might prove rewarding.

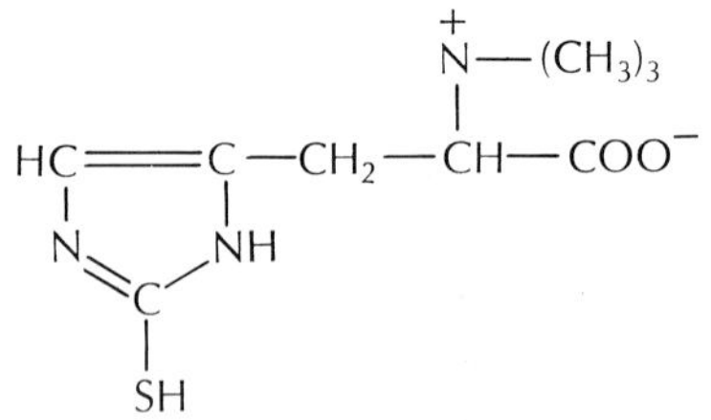

FIGURE 8-3. Structure of ergothioneine.

Adenosine 3′, 5′-monophosphate (Cyclic AMP)

Primarily through the work of Sutherland and his associates, a variety of hormonal actions are now known to be mediated by cyclic AMP. Thus the epinephrine-stimulated glycogenolysis in skeletal muscle, the secretion of insulin, lipolysis in fat cells, and the release of thyroid stimulating hormone, all appear to be under the control of this cyclic nucleotide. In the central nervous system there is as yet no direct evidence that links cyclic AMP with brain function, but some recent reports provide a strong suggestion that a relationship does exist. The current evidence may be summarized as follows:

1. Of all mammalian tissues examined, the brain has the highest activity of adenyl cyclase, the enzyme that catalyzes the synthesis of cyclic AMP from ATP. In addition, the activity of cyclic 3′, 5′-nucleotide phosphodiesterase, the enzyme which hydrolyzes cyclic AMP, is also higher in brain than in any other tissue.

2. Adenyl cyclase appears to be localized in synaptic membranes.

3. The level of cyclic AMP in brain slices is increased by electrical stimulation.

4. The addition of norepinephrine, serotonin, and histamine to respiring brain slices increases the concentration of cyclic AMP in the slices.

5. Caffeine and theophylline, which are mild central nervous system stimulants, inhibit phosphodiesterase.

6. A cyclic AMP-dependent protein kinase has been discovered in brain.

7. When cyclic AMP or norepinephrine is applied microelectrophoretically to the cerebellum the discharge frequency of the Purkinje cells is reduced. This effect is enhanced by theophylline.

Thus, there is moderately compelling evidence that adenosine 3′, 5′-monophosphate plays some role in the central nervous system which further experimentation should define.

SELECTED REFERENCES

Clark, W. G., and G. Ungar (1964). Histamine and the nervous system. *Fed. Proc. 23*, 1095.

Crossland, J., G. N. Woodruff, and J. F. Mitchell (1964). Identity of the cerebellar factor. *Nature 203*, 1388.

Euler, U. S. von, and R. Eliasson (1967). *Prostaglandins*. Academic Press, New York.

Haefely, W., and A. Hürlimann (1962). Substance P, a highly active naturally occurring polypeptide. *Experientia 18*, 297.

Horton, W. W. (1969). Hypotheses on physiological roles of prostaglandins. *Physiol. Rev. 49*, 122.

Krnjevic, K. K. (1965). Action of drugs on single neurons in cerebral cortex. *Brit. Med. Bull. 21*, 10.

Lembeck, F., Zeller, E. A. (1962). Substance P: a polypeptide of possible physiological significance, especially within the nervous system. *Int. Rev. Neurobiology 4*, 159.

Rocha E Silva, M. (1966). Histamine, its chemistry, metabolism and pqhysiological and pharmacological actions. *Handbuch der Experimentellen Pharmakologie 18*, 1.

Sutherland, E. W., G. A. Robison, and R. W. Butcher (1968). Some aspects of the biological role of adenosine 3', 5'-monophosphate (cyclic AMP). *Circulation 37*, 279.

9 | Cellular Mechanisms in Memory and Learning

AT THE PRESENT time no one has shown unequivocally a causal relation between a change in cell structure or function and learning. In reality this sentence is all that is necessary to discuss this topic. Nevertheless we feel compelled to examine the theories and the experimental findings in this field for two reasons. First, this area comes under the domain of neuropharmacology since drugs have been used both directly to stimulate learning and indirectly as tools to explore molecular mechanisms which may be involved. Second, there is a great deal of appeal and excitement attached to this topic; thus we feel an obligation to prevent the impressionable and the romantically inclined from being seduced into this glamorous field before they know the pitfalls.

Before proceeding further it is necessary to define some terms that are encountered. "Memory" may be defined as the storage and retrieval of sensory information. Many investigators refer to "short-term memory" which is likened to reverberatory circuits and which operationally may be ablated by coma, anesthesia, or electroconvulsive therapy. "Long-term memory" refers to the consolidation of information with long-term storage and has been suggested to involve protein synthesis. It is still not clear if there is a sequential progression of short-term into long-term memory or if two different mechanisms are concerned. By "learning" we mean the modification of behavior through experience. However, since this simple definition would not exclude phenomena such as synaptic facilitation, post-tetanic potentiation, sensory adaptation, or fatigue, some investigators prefer a more detailed definition. They define learning as "a modification of a stimulus-response complex which involves the afferent nervous system and which in whole animals results in a new favorable adaptation." It is obvious that memory and learning are related, but memory is only a part of learning since learning infers a change in performance due to a gain in our understanding.

There are two other terms we should consider. "Sensitization" refers to an augmentation of a response to the conditioned stimulus. This means that the system becomes more efficient in being able to perceive or transmit the sensory stimuli and evoke the appropriate motor response. The opposite of sensitization is "habituation" which implies a progressive decrease in response to a given sensory signal. That this suppression is not due to a general fatigue of an organism may be shown by changing the stimulus and noting a return of a full response.

Formulating Theories on Memory and Learning

Theories on memory and learning existed long before the anatomy of the nervous system was known. However, once the neuron was recognized as the basic functional unit of the nervous system, Ramon y Cajal was among the first to postulate that the process of learning involves structural changes at synaptic contacts. He apparently based this view upon the fact that with maturation of the nerve cells the dendritic trees sprouted spines as a sign of their complex maturation. He recognized that the synaptic contact was the primary site of communication between nerve cells and seemed to be a logical point at which to alter the efficiency of the information passage. Furthermore, he believed that electrical activity of one cell would favor the development of connections to a second cell, and thus that the availability of sensory inputs activating certain parts of the system would favor the development of new connections to other portions of the system.

The essential feature of this "specific connection" view of

learning is that the experienced input modified the output by making a change either in the efficiency of the existing connection or by making more or newer connections between specific nervous cells. The opposite view was taken by many American psychologists during the early part of the twentieth century. They held that specific pathways or pre-existing connections between nerve cells had little or nothing to do with the learning process, and emphasized instead changes in nerve cell activity related to the external environment of the cell: possibly the extracellular space, possibly the electrical gradients from one portion of the cortex across another. In general this "field" theory depended upon influences much larger than any single cell or single group of cells. While the comprehension of this "field" or "global" model of learning presents many difficulties, the greatest one perhaps is that it is nearly impossible to subject the theory to experimental testing. On the other hand, the cellular or connectionistic viewpoint of learning can be subjected to modern electrophysiological and morphological techniques.

Morphological Experiments

If activity within a defined nerve-to-nerve connection is able to influence the subsequent transmission through that same connection, then one might expect to find morphological variations associated with use and disuse. Numerous experiments along this line of investigation have been attempted, but the results offer little in the way of concrete support. The failure may be due to the fact that over-use or under-use are often produced by highly nonphysiological techniques such as cutting muscles, cutting nerves, or prolonged electrical stimulation. Another negative aspect may be that the systems involved are not necessarily those at which plastic or dynamic structural properties exist. However, even within the central nervous system, in areas such as the visual cortex or lateral geniculate (a relay nucleus of the visual system), it has been nearly impossible to demonstrate long-term changes in either electrical conduction or morphological connections with variations in activity through the visual system. With the electron microscope it may be possible to use specific staining reactions to quantitate the number and size of specialized synaptic contacts and thus to obtain a more objective measurement than can be made with empirical silver staining techniques which are often hit or miss in their resolution of nerve cells.

The types of experiments which have been reported center upon the neuromuscular junction or on other forms of reinner-vated peripheral junctions such as sympathetic ganglia or other muscle preparations. Here it can be shown that when the muscle is kept at rest, or when the nerve is cut and the transmission across the junction is reduced, the muscle develops increased receptive-ness for the neurotransmitter, namely, acetylcholine. This would suggest that disuse affects the junction by making it more sensi-tive to transmission. This is the opposite of the more commonly expressed view that usage favors the efficiency of transmission whereas nonusage impairs it. In the central nervous system, these two opposing views have not been studied in clearcut experiments and no final answer can be given at present. When animals are deprived of their visual imput by closing both eyes at birth be-fore the first perception of sensory stimuli, there are no changes in neurophysiological conduction of signals when both eyes are subsequently opened. However, more complex changes can be seen: if one eye is kept closed and the other allowed to develop normally, the normally occurring bilateral interaction between the eyes cannot be subsequently demonstrated. Such findings fail to discriminate between activity required for development and activity affecting efficiency of usage.

CELLULAR MODELS FOR LEARNING EXPERIMENTS

The experimental tasks required to determine the nature of the cellular processes underlying the changes which occur with learning constitute one of the most difficult problem areas in sci-ence. It is essential to uncover a neuronal system in which expe-rience, in the form of electrical stimulation, chemical stimulation, or natural stimulation (such as light or sound) can be shown to induce permanent changes in the conduction of impulses and which would thus offer a cellular model for the learning mechanism. Such a model has not yet been described.

However, numerous experiments have been reported (see the review by Kandel and Spencer) in which scientists have attempted to break down the behavioral analogues of the learning procedure, as based on the conditioned stimulus, condition avoidance, or operant types of learning situations. These experiments have indicated clearly that prolonged types of physiological change can be induced by activity. All cells do not exhibit these changes, but only particular cells such as giant neurons in molluscan ganglia or pacemaker type cells in simpler systems. When the transmembrane potential level is analyzed during these experiments, the plastic or experimentally induced changes in activity do not appear to arise from changes induced in the postsynaptic cell, its transmembrane resistance or capacitance, or the spike generating system. Therefore, whatever the changes are, they appear to be either within the synapse or on the presynaptic side of the system involved in the conditioning or learning. The mechanisms which have been suggested involve hyperpolarization of the presynaptic terminals by activity in the conditioning system: this hyperpolarization results in an enhanced effect through the test circuit when it is effectively stimulated and could cause an increased response to the conditioning. The effects need not involve two different circuits since prolonged stimulation of a single monosynaptic pathway can also result in enhanced effects of that pathway simply due to post-tetanic hyperpolarization. Such effects can last for hours. In similar fashion, the suggestion has been made that habituation could result from depression in the test pathway due to prolonged activity in the conditioning pathways which could in turn arise from enhancement of inhibitory postsynaptic potentials.

The problem, however, in relation to mammalian learning, is that experiments on molluscan ganglia, or even headless insect ganglia, confirm only the possibility that prolonged, possibly permanent, changes in the relationship of transmission between one or more cells in the circuit can be demonstrated. They do not tell us that these types of plastic change can exist in higher forms or that they are the only possible mechanisms by which plastic change may occur. Therefore, we must hope that neuronal systems for studying the learning process in animals more closely related to the mammal can be uncovered and that their mechanisms can be studied with the same types of cellular techniques.

Until a system for such study evolves, it appears fruitless to attempt to analyze with the electron microscope the possible plastic changes occurring in the mammalian central nervous system. Although we can suggest numerous possible mechanisms for such plastic change (such as increased size of specialized synaptic contacts, increased size of dendritic spines, increased numbers of synaptic vesicles), none of these changes can be documented meaningfully until we are able to identify a neuronal circuit in which a defined physiological function has been altered by the factors of use, disuse, or some other equivalent of the learning experience situation. The numerous variables involved in the size, number, and density of synaptic contacts for any particular nerve cell of the mammalian central nervous system is as yet poorly defined, and until such variables can be eliminated and until a specific circuit can be studied by both physiology and fine structure, an electron microscopic study on the learning process would seem to be much like the proverbial hunt for a needle in a haystack, except that in this case the needle may not exist at all.

Concurrent with electrophysiological approaches to the study of memory and learning, a number of neuroscientists have attempted to uncover molecular mechanisms in behavior using drugs as tools. We will now consider this biochemical approach.

BIOCHEMICAL EXPERIMENTATION ON LEARNING AND MEMORY

As Kandell and Spencer point out, biochemical investigations on cellular mechanisms involved in memory and learning can be classified into four approaches:

1. *Facilitation.* Numerous investigators have used a variety of drugs in an attempt to increase the rate of learning. Agents that

have been used include strychnine, picrotoxin, magnesium pemoline, RNA, amphetamine, and K^+. Positive, negative, and inconclusive results have been obtained with this approach. Such a range is almost predictable in view of the enormous number of variables involved: the type of drug used, the route of administration, the dose, the type of task involved in learning, and the strain, sex, and age of organisms that are tested. To these complexities we must also add the time element in the experiment, that is, giving the drug before learning or after learning, testing immediately or later. Even if a positive result were obtained, the effect of the drug could still be completely nonspecific and bear no primary relationship to the learning process but only to the rate of processing of information, for example, by an arousal effect on the animal.

2. *Transfer.* This line of investigation involves the administration of brain extracts from trained animals to untrained ones (referred to as naïve). These naïve recipients are then compared with control animals to see if their ability to learn the task is facilitated. Planaria (flatworms) were among the first organisms to be used in these experiments since not only are they cannibalistic, but they can be bisected and each half will regenerate the lost half-torso complete with rudimentary nervous system. There are two major problems with these planaria experiments: first, an enormous number of unknown variables must exist, since it has been difficult for one laboratory to duplicate results from another; second, the more basic unresolved question, do planaria learn? The known variables that require rigid control are the species and the source of the worms, the kind of training they receive, the amount and type of food they are given, the kind of shock that is administered, the time of day the experiments are done, the amount of handling the worms receive, the condition of their trough (planaria leave slime trails), the ion concentration of the water, and the light sensitivity of the worms. In addition, in early experiments the bias of the investigator was not controlled.

Mice and rats have also been used in transfer experiments.

Ungar injected mice with brain extracts from rats that were habituated to sound and stated that the mice lost their startle response to the same sound stimulus. It was also reported that these mice responded normally to air-puff whereas mice that were injected with brain extracts from rats habituated to air-puff had a decreased response to air-puff but not to sound. Other experiments involved Y-maze training in which the rats in order to escape a shock were trained to run into the lighted arm of the maze. Brain extracts from the trained rats were then injected i.p. into mice and the mice were tested for their ability to escape the shock by running to the light. In these and similar experiments statistically significant positive results were observed and the investigators claimed to have exhibited a transfer of learning.

In all these transfer experiments it should be no surprise to the reader to learn that some difficulty has been encountered in attempting to duplicate the results in other laboratories. On theoretical grounds alone it would appear improbable since (a) the injected material in which the information is presumed to be encoded in a biopolymer such as a protein or nucleic acid must pass the blood-brain barrier intact. (b) This macromolecule must seek out the precise neuronal network that is concerned with the stimulus-specific learned behavior. (c) This macromolecule must then somehow be incorporated as an intact molecule.

On the more pragmatic side, the major criticism in these experiments is that there are innumerable variables in training and testing. Further, what is referred to as a simple T- or Y-maze, one of the commonly used tests, is far from simple according to experimental psychologists.

3. *Interruption.* Procedures for interfering with the consolidation of information generally involve the intracranial injection of antibiotics that disrupt protein synthesis. Puromycin, cycloheximide, and acetoxycycloheximide are the popular agents that have been employed. Some similar experiments have also been done with nucleic acid inhibitors such as actinomycin D, which inhibits DNA-dependent RNA polymerase, and 8-azaguanine, which is incorporated into nucleic acids. Both of these agents

will, of course, subsequently interfere with protein biosynthesis.

For an individual not working in this area it is difficult to relate a coherent account of these experiments with protein inhibitors. Not only are the experimental conditions constantly varied but interpretations change with each publication and the committed investigators in this area are not entirely in agreement on acceptable criteria.

If we take experiments with puromycin as an example these difficulties will be readily apparent. Puromycin, an analogue of transfer RNA, blocks protein synthesis by disrupting polysomes; it is released from polysomes as a peptidyl-puromycin. Flexner and Flexner injected puromycin into both temporal lobes of mice which had been trained in a T-maze. In their initial report they found no effect on memory but in a subsequent paper they showed that whereas short-term memory was unimpaired, long-term memory was blocked. In a succeeding paper, the Flexners then showed that the memory could be restored by an intracerebral injection of saline. More recently they observed the saline injections were ineffective in restoring memory if the puromycin was given either before or immediately after training. Most recently, they reported that if instead of injecting saline two days after the administration of puromycin they wait five or ten days, then the saline restores memory.

With respect to the mechanism of action of puromycin, the Flexners suggest that the memory block is due to the presence of peptidyl-puromycin in the brain.

Cohen and Barondes found that cycloheximide prevented the effect of puromycin in blocking memory in mice. Cohen and Erwin demonstrated that the intracranial injection of puromycin produced seizure-like EEG changes in the hippocampal region. By contrast, cycloheximide had no such effect. Cohen and Barondes later found that this seizure effect of puromycin could, in fact, be blocked by previous administration of cycloheximide. Further, the anticonvulsant diphenylhydantoin not only blocked the abnormal EEG effect of puromycin but also prevented the inhibiting effect of puromycin on memory.

Cohen and Barondes found that acetoxycycloheximide injected intracerebrally to mice trained for light-dark discrimination produced no loss in memory for up to three hours after the training session. However, six hours after training, memory was impaired in the mice trained to a 9 out of 10 correct response criterion. If training was then continued to a criterion of 15 out of 16 correct responses, there was no amnesic effect of the drug. That is to say, overtraining abolishes the drug effect. In another experiment these authors found that when mice that were trained to discriminate between left and right, rather than light-dark as above, were injected with acetoxycycloheximide, no impairment of memory was observed when they were trained to the usual criterion of 9 out of 10 correct responses.

Agranoff trained goldfish to swim over a hurdle toward a light in order to escape a shock, and found that puromycin, as well as acetoxycycloheximide and actinomycin D, blocks this long-term memory: no effect on short-term memory by these agents was noted. Cytosine arabinoside, a DNA synthesis inhibitor, had no effect on short- or long-term memory.

What can one conclude from these experiments with agents that block protein synthesis? First of all it is clear with puromycin that one is dealing with an agent that does more than inhibit protein synthesis. Although no other effects of the other protein inhibitors have been reported as yet, it is more than probable that they occur. The student must be aware that there is no such thing as a "pure" drug that has only one biochemical action. There is an aphorism that every drug has two actions: the one you know about and the one you don't. It can, therefore, be concluded that it is too early to make conclusions about the relationship between protein synthesis and memory. That such an association may exist is not denied: it just is not yet proven. Second, it is also clear that the complexities in the type of training given, the training period, the timing of the injections of drugs, the kind of drug, the site of injection, and a host of other variables are such that meaningful experiments are difficult. Finally, on a more personal note, it is not without considerable irritation that one reviews the literature on this subject because of the plethora of premature publications that manifest questionable critical judgment.

4. *Correlation* between learning and biochemical changes in cells. This approach is exemplified by the work of Hydén and his colleagues. In a succession of studies, animals were either rotated on a turntable, trained to balance on a steel wire, or trained to transfer handedness (e.g. to use the right paw instead of the left). Then, the biochemistry of cells from the "appropriate" area of the brain in experimental and control animals was determined. In the rotation and steel wire experiments, neurons and glia were dissected out of Dieters' nucleus; in the transfer of handedness, cells from the 5th and 6th layers of the cortex were removed. In these experiments Hydén found changes in the base pair ratios of RNA, an increase in the amount of RNA, increase in the activity of some enzymes and in total protein. Similar but not identical changes were found both in the neurons and the glia that were examined.

These experiments have been severely criticized:

1. In the dissection of neurons and glia there is contamination of one by the other. Moreover, in neurons only the perikaryon is dissected out and the remaining neuronal elements, in particular the dendritic branches which also contain RNA, are left behind.

2. The cells involved in the specific learning procedure have not been mapped out so that Hydén cannot possibly correlate learning with a biochemical change in the function of the cell or group of cells. Also the state of the cells after learning is unknown. That is, for example, did the cells taken from Dieters' nucleus of animals which were rotated have an increased or decreased rate of discharge, i.e. were they activated or depressed?

3. No attempt was made to look at the condition of dissected neurons either electrophysiologically or with an electron microscope to assess their viability.

4. Since local circulatory changes sometimes accompany stimulation of neuronal pathways *in vivo*, the biochemical

changes observed by Hydén and his group may reflect increased transport of substrates rather than an association with learning.

5. If indeed new RNA were being formed it would be extremely difficult to determine it in the presence of a large mass of genetically determined, i.e. fixed, RNA.

In reviewing the variety of approaches that have been taken in the study of the mechanisms of memory and learning, the advantages of using simple neural preparations rather than whole animals become obvious. For example, the headless cockroach preparation appears most promising. Here a conditioned avoidance response of a leg attached to the prothoracic ganglion is used along with a yoked control preparation. The preparation "learned" to avoid a shock by retraction of the leg. It has been shown that cycloheximide can block this "learning" (though this agent may also affect performance rather than learning). Since in this preparation one can map out the motor cells within the ganglion and their connections to the leg muscles, it may be possible to establish a specific association between protein synthesis and learning.

At the present time one can only state that protein and RNA synthesis may occur along with learning but the experiment has yet to be designed that explicitly relates these two events. The somewhat chaotic condition of this field is due not only to an inordinate amount of dross that has been presented but to monistic interpretations of data. Caveat emptor.

Flexner, J. B., and L. B. Flexner (1969). Studies in memory: evidence for a widespread memory trace in the neocortex after the suppression of recent memory by puromycin. *Proc. Nat. Acad. Sci. 62*, 729.

Glassman, E. (1969). The biochemistry of learning. An evaluation of the role of RNA and protein. *Ann. Rev. Biochem. 38*, 605.

Kandel, E. R., and W. A. Spencer (1968). Cellular neurophysiological approaches in the study of learning. *Physiol. Rev. 48*, 65.

Quarton, G. C., T. Melnechuk, and F. O. Schmitt (1967). *The neurosciences—A Study Program.* Rockefeller Univ. Press, New York.

Index